TEEN PROBLEMS

TEENS AND DEPRESSION

By A.W. Buckey

ReferencePoint Press®

San Diego, CA

ReferencePoint Press®

Printed in the United States

For more information, contact:
ReferencePoint Press, Inc.
PO Box 27779
San Diego, CA 92198
www.ReferencePointPress.com

Content Consultant: Lindsey B. Stone, PhD, Assistant Professor of Psychology, Christopher Newport University

LIBRARY OF CONGRESS CATALOGING-IN-PUBLICATION DATA

Names: Buckey, A. W., author.
Title: Teens and depression / by A.W. Buckey.
Description: San Diego, CA : ReferencePoint Press, [2021] | Series: Teen problems | Includes bibliographical references and index. | Audience: Grades 10-12
Identifiers: LCCN 2020003705 (print) | LCCN 2020003706 (eBook) | ISBN 9781682829592 (hardcover) | ISBN 9781682829608 (eBook)
Subjects: LCSH: Depression in adolescence--Juvenile literature.
Classification: LCC RJ506.D4 B83 2021 (print) | LCC RJ506.D4 (eBook) | DDC 616.85/2700835--dc23
LC record available at https://lccn.loc.gov/2020003705
LC eBook record available at https://lccn.loc.gov/2020003706

CONTENTS

INTRODUCTION

THE NAMELESS PROBLEM

Starting middle school can feel like entering an unfamiliar world. There are new people, new rules, and a new place to be every day. That's how it felt for ten-year-old Naomi Ekperigin on her first day at the Dalton School in New York City. She was with a small group of totally new classmates, and she was one of the few black students in a mostly white school. Ekperigin was a good student and liked doing well in her classes. She made her classmates laugh and discovered her talent for comedy. Still, middle school was a lonely time for her. Now a comedian, Ekperigin reflected on the history of her mental health struggles in an interview with podcast host John Moe. She remembers crying every day her first year at the new school. "I just felt so out of place," Ekperigin says.[1]

Over the next few years, Ekperigin continued to succeed academically. But her feelings of sadness and isolation deepened. Like most teenagers, Ekperigin had new friendships

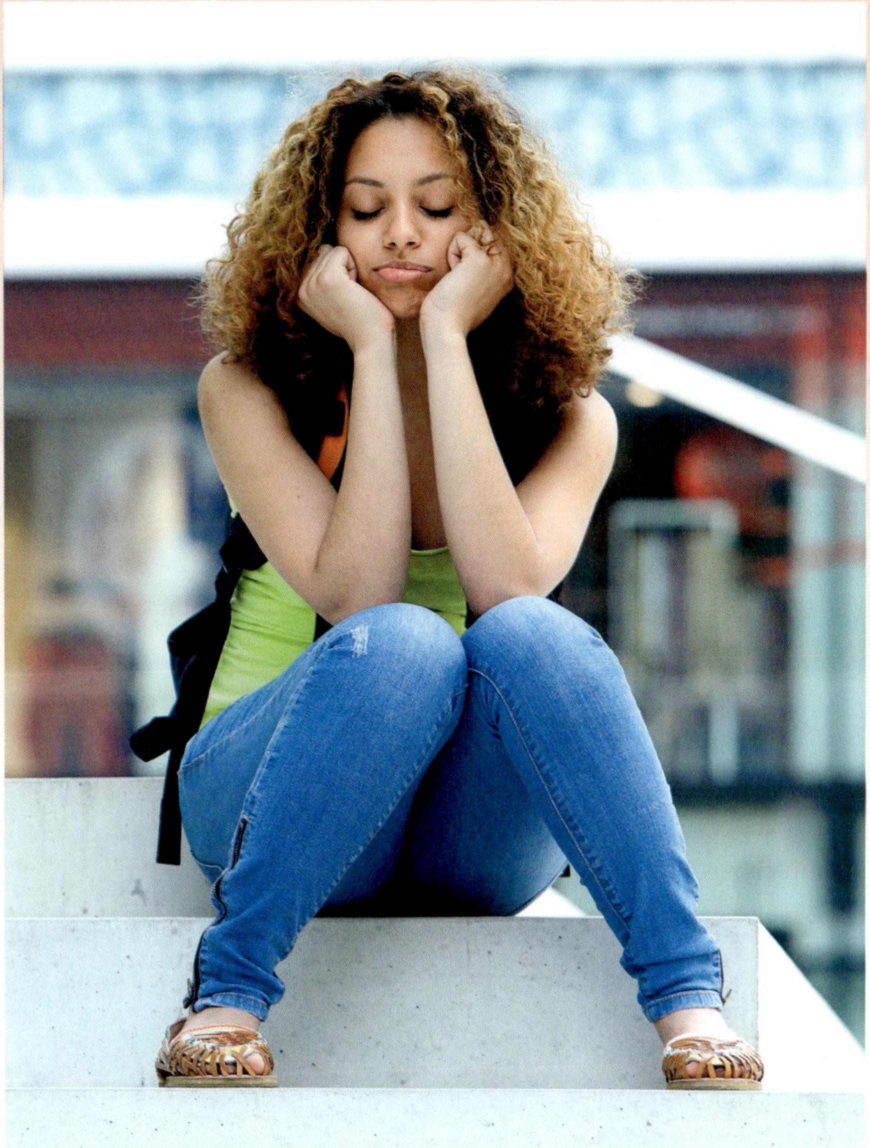

Some teens struggle to identify how they are feeling. A diagnosis may help them give a name to their feelings.

and crushes to navigate. But the normal social drama of high school life felt devastating. Many teenagers are familiar with constant criticism through social media and social interactions.

But Ekperigin remembers that a simple thing like feeling rejected by a friend "would be the . . . reason to cry and stay in the house and not leave and not talk to anybody for days."[2]

During this time, Ekperigin was also struggling with her relationship with her father. He had disappeared from her life for several years. Around the time she started middle school, he reentered her life. However, their relationship was distant and awkward. Ekperigin felt rejected by her father. She believes that the pain of her lost relationship with her dad made her more sensitive to rejection from peers and boys: "I would take any rejection as the fundamental proof that I was unlovable and I was inadequate," Ekperigin said.[3] Even happy times were hard to truly enjoy. "I could never take full joy in anything that was happening."[4] Her feelings of disconnection from others seemed impossible to escape, coloring the way that she looked at her life.

> "I could never take full joy in anything that was happening."[4]
>
> —*Naomi Ekperigin, comedian*

When Ekperigin got to college in Connecticut, her feelings of sadness and rejection were harder to handle. She felt overwhelmed being away from home: "Everything just felt like it was so much more intense, so much more of a pressure cooker," Ekperigin says, reflecting on that time.[5] To cope with her emotions, Ekperigin turned to self-harm. She began cutting herself. Ekperigin knew she needed help. She sought out a mental health counselor on her college campus. The counselor referred her to a psychiatrist, or a doctor who specializes in mental illnesses. After her first year of college, Ekperigin's struggles finally got a name: she was suffering from depression. Ekperigin began seeing her doctor regularly and taking medications for her illness. It was a relief for her to finally have words to describe what she was going through: "I love a diagnosis," Ekperigin jokes.[6]

> "Everything just felt like it was so much more intense, so much more of a pressure cooker."[5]
>
> —*Naomi Ekperigin, comedian*

Even though Naomi Ekperigin spent years feeling alone, her story is common. As many as 20 percent of American teens may suffer from major depression, also known as depression. Depression in teens can have many causes, and the symptoms of depression may change over time. One common thread in stories of depression, however, is that the feelings suffered go far beyond simple sadness. Depression takes the energy and joy from its sufferers, and without treatment its effects can last for years or a lifetime. With treatment and understanding, however, there is hope for teens with depression and their loved ones.

CHAPTER ONE

WHAT IS TEEN DEPRESSION?

The word *depression* can mean any kind of low point or period of reduced activity. People often use the word *depressed* to describe someone who is sad or seems less active or energetic than usual. Depression is considered a mood disorder, in which people experience an extreme change of mood, which makes them interact with their world in a different way. Depression has a few other medical names. In the United States, health care professionals use a book called the *Diagnostic and Statistical Manual of Mental Disorders* (*DSM*) to describe and diagnose mental illnesses. The most recent version of this book, the *DSM-5*, lists eight different depressive disorders, or mental illnesses that feature low moods and reduced ability to function. The most common of these disorders is called major depressive disorder. Other terms for major depressive disorder include clinical depression and major depression.

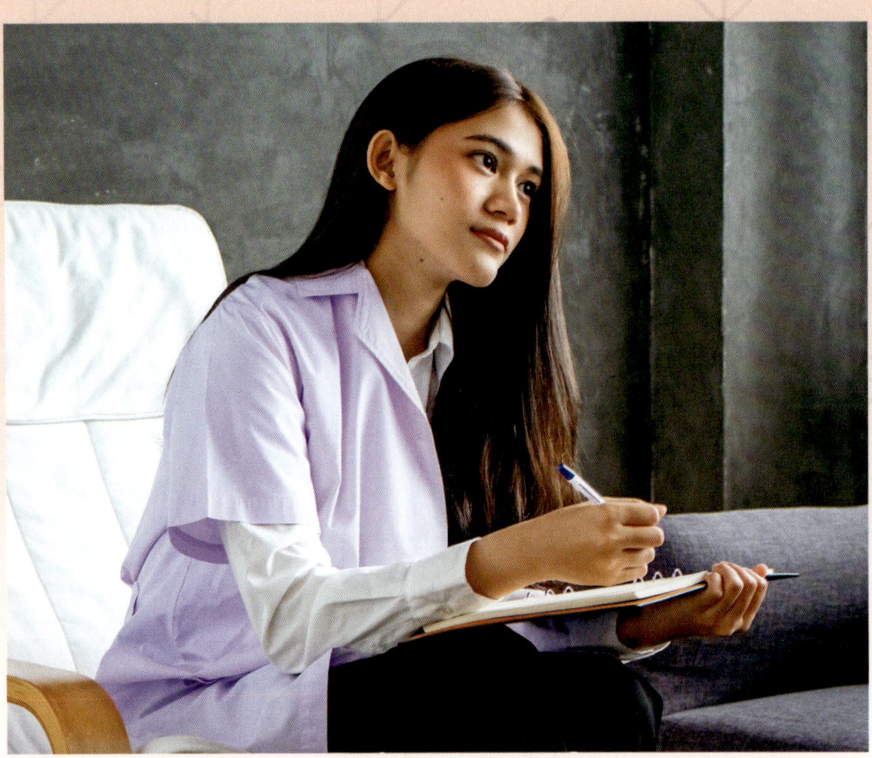

Health care professionals use the *DSM-5* to diagnose depression. Professionals study someone's symptoms to determine whether the patient may have one of the eight depressive disorders.

MAJOR DEPRESSIVE DISORDER

Mental illnesses are defined and diagnosed differently than diseases, such as the flu, or physical injuries, such as broken bones. Mental illnesses are syndromes, which means they are defined by their symptoms, not their causes. Physical illnesses often have a single cause; for example, the disease malaria is caused by a parasite entering the blood through a mosquito's bite. Not everyone who gets malaria has the exact same symptoms, but they all contract the disease the same way.

In contrast, depression can be caused by a variety of factors, and two people may become depressed for different reasons. It is the suffering, and not the reasons behind it, that defines depression. This suffering manifests in different ways.

Depression symptoms have a common link: they negatively affect the mind, spirit, and body. However, this lowering of mood and spirits can feel and look very different from person to person and over time. For this reason, depression is defined by a cluster of symptoms. Depressed people show many, but usually not all, of the symptoms of depression over an extended period.

The *DSM-5* outlines nine key symptoms of major depressive disorder. To receive a depression diagnosis, a person must have at least five of the nine symptoms. People with depression may suffer from a depressed or sad mood most of the day and may be uninterested in or unable to enjoy most parts of their lives.

Physical symptoms of depression include appetite loss and significant weight loss or gain; either insomnia, which is the inability to sleep, or hypersomnia, which is sleeping too much; physical restlessness or slowness; and lasting tiredness or lack of energy. People with depression also may experience changes in their thinking. Depression can cause people to feel persistent, inappropriate guilt and feelings of worthlessness. They may experience "brain fog" and not be able to concentrate or make decisions. In addition, depressed people may suffer from suicidal ideation, where they think about suicide or make plans to take their own lives.

In order to be diagnosed with depression, one of the five symptoms experienced must be either suffering from a sad mood most of the day or not finding enjoyment in most parts of life. In addition, the symptoms must continue almost every day for a period of two weeks. These guidelines are designed to help mental health professionals tell the difference between a low period and the start of a disorder.

It's common for people with depression to experience rumination, or obsessive negative thoughts. Depressed teens may find themselves thinking the same hopeless, negative thoughts about themselves and the world over and over again. Elise Jamison, who was diagnosed with depression at fourteen, explained, "Depression is the dark emptiness you feel that makes you believe you can contribute nothing to anyone or anything. You feel like your life means nothing to anyone."[7] These thoughts can have a severe, damaging impact on someone's mood.

> "Depression is the dark emptiness you feel that makes you believe you can contribute nothing to anyone or anything. You feel like your life means nothing to anyone."[7]
>
> *—Elise Jamison, high schooler with depression*

Sometimes, teen depression goes unrecognized. A stereotype about teens is that they are moody and emotional, withdrawing from others during difficult times. It's true that puberty and the physical and mental changes of the teen years can have strong effects on mood. But depression is much more than normal emotional ups and downs. A depressed teen suffers from low moods regardless of what is going on around them. The depressed feelings are outside their control. Psychiatrists Patrick Kelly and Francis Mark Mondimore point out, "Seriously depressed adolescents can't 'shake off' their mood states or get their minds off their troubles by concentrating on school or sports or friends."[8] If they do experience a reprieve from low moods, it is often brief.

> "Seriously depressed adolescents can't 'shake off' their mood states or get their minds off their troubles by concentrating on school or sports or friends."[8]
>
> *—Dr. Patrick Kelly and Dr. Francis Mark Mondimore, psychiatrists*

Another common depressive disorder is called persistent depressive disorder, or dysthymia. Persistent depressive disorder is less intense but longer-lasting than major depressive disorder. According to the *DSM-5*, "Individuals with persistent depressive disorder describe their mood as sad or 'down in the dumps.'"[9] People with persistent depressive disorder suffer from low moods, but they need to have only two of the symptoms of depression. These symptoms must last for at least a year for teens to get a persistent depressive disorder diagnosis.

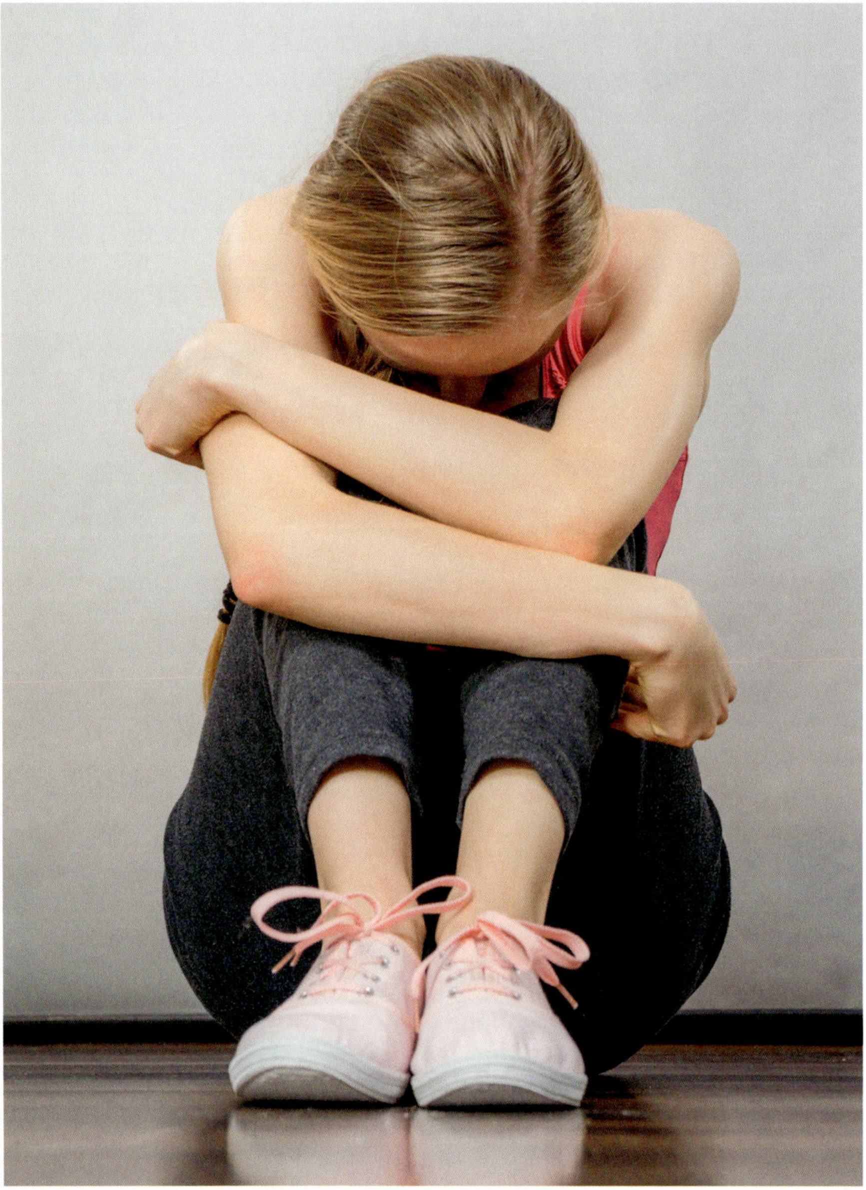

Teens may have persistent depressive disorder if they have felt sad for a year or longer. This feeling of sadness is not something they can control.

Both major depressive disorder and persistent depressive disorder are commonly known as depression, and a person can suffer from either or both disorders at different times.

THE HISTORY OF DEPRESSION

Human beings have recognized the existence of depression since ancient times. Ancient Greek philosophers called depression "melancholia," and the word *melancholy* still means sadness or depressed mood. Many cultures believed that depression was caused by imbalances in the body. Ancient Hindu scriptures theorized that depression was caused by disturbances in invisible bodily energies called doshas. Medieval European medicine saw depression as the result of imbalanced fluids in the body. Some early Christians believed depression stemmed from internal demons, which led priests to perform exorcisms, or the dispelling of demons from the body.

In Europe in the 1700s and 1800s, two schools of thought argued over the causes of mental disorders like depression. Some doctors, like mental hospital founder Henry Maudsley, believed that mental illness had a biological cause. He also believed mental disorders were heritable, or passed down from parents to children. However, the 1800s was also the time of the birth of new psychological theories. Sigmund Freud was an Austrian doctor who invented a treatment called psychoanalysis. In this process, patients talked with a doctor in one-on-one sessions to uncover and change their patterns of thinking. Freud believed that depression was the result of unconscious anger and aggression turned inward. He thought depressed people

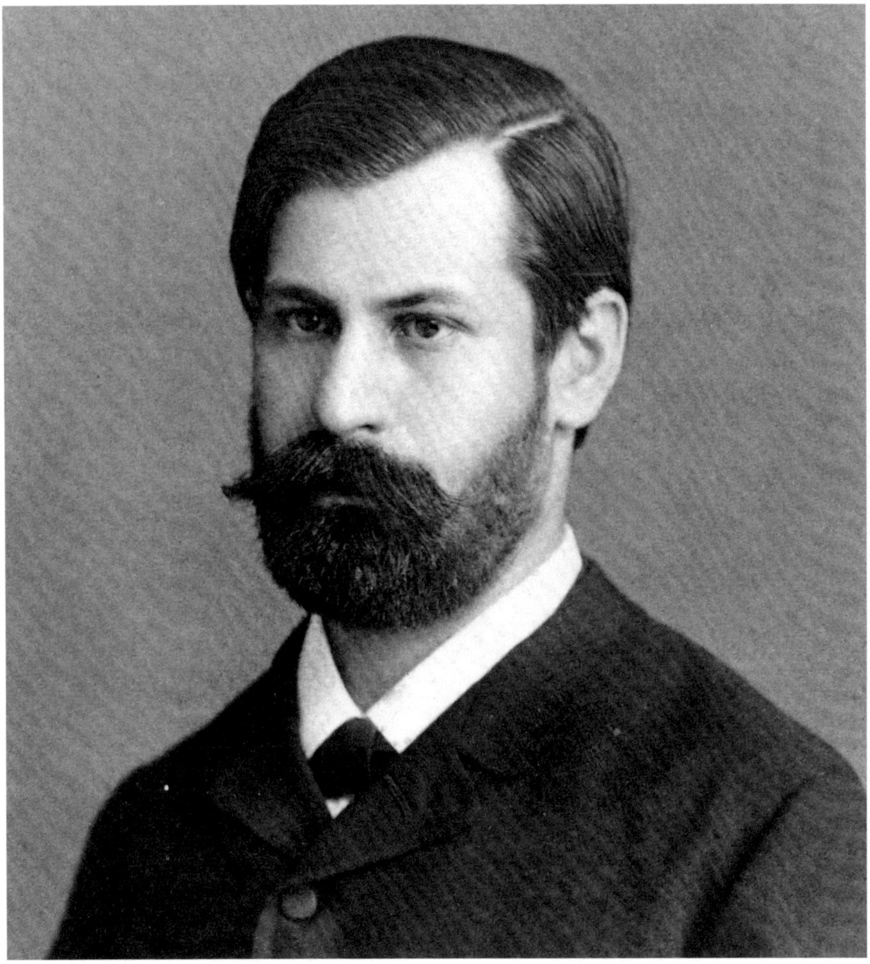

Sigmund Freud was the founder of psychoanalysis. Psychoanalysis is now a technique used to treat depression.

became angry and distressed by loss, and they dealt with anger by directing the hate and guilt at themselves. Although Freud's theories were not based on scientific testing, they became very influential.

In the mid-twentieth century, many scientists and researchers investigated how depression works in the brain. Instead of

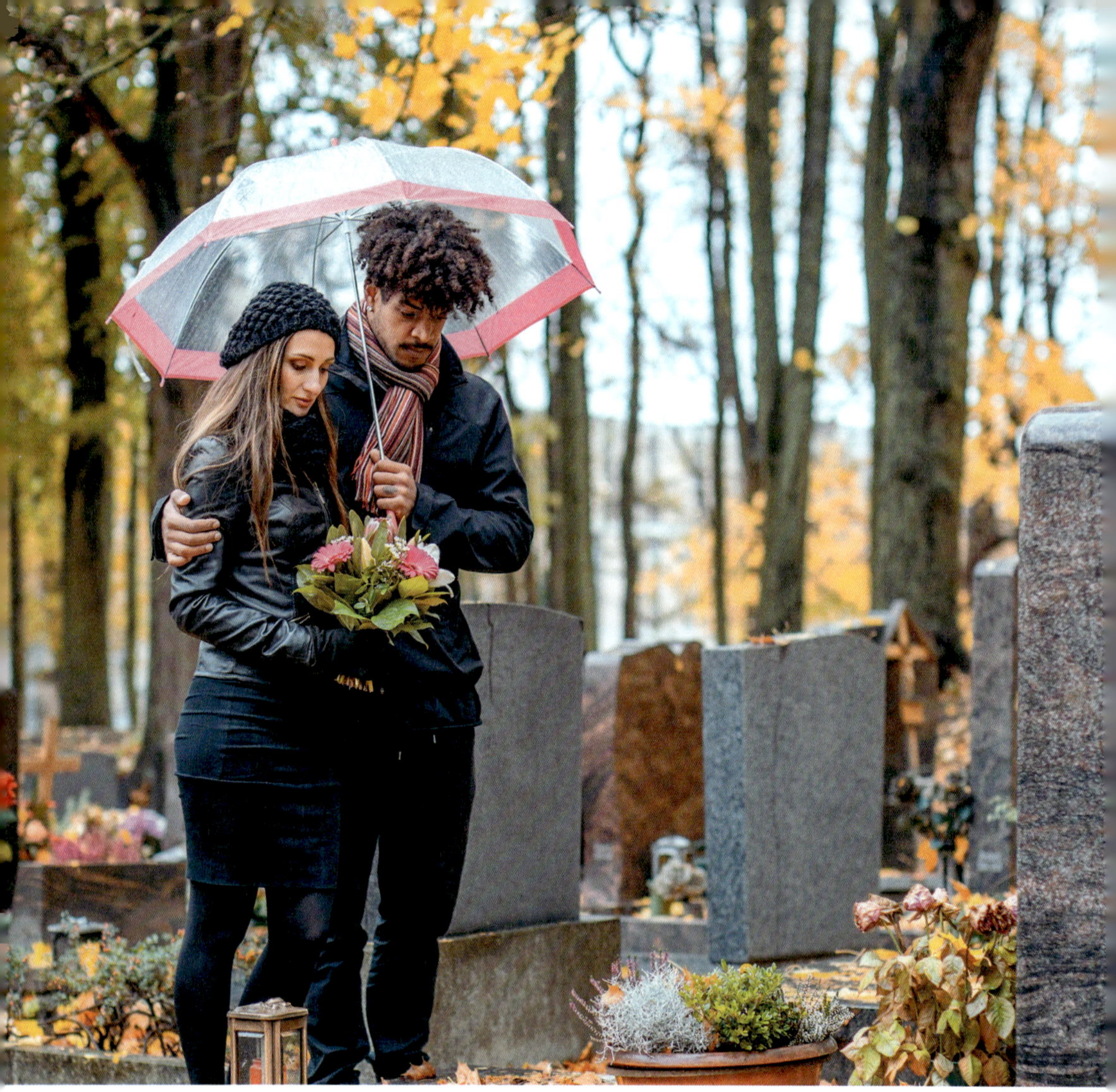

Stressful life events, such as the death of a loved one, can cause depression. Doctors may also refer to this as stress response syndrome.

imbalances in bodily forces, these scientists looked for imbalances in the chemicals of the brain that might cause depressive symptoms. The conception of depression as a disorder caused by chemical, biological factors is known as the biomedical model.

Today, mental health professionals acknowledge that depression can have many causes per individual case. According to Harvard Medical School, "There are many possible causes of depression, including faulty mood regulation by the brain, genetic vulnerability, stressful life events, medications, and medical problems."[10]

> "There are many possible causes of depression, including faulty mood regulation by the brain, genetic vulnerability, stressful life events, medications, and medical problems."[10]
>
> —*Harvard Medical School*

HOW DEPRESSION IS DIAGNOSED

Mental health professionals can diagnose depression in teens. There are several different professions that specialize in diagnosing and treating mental disorders. Psychiatrists are one example, as well as psychologists and social workers, who are trained differently but work with similar patients. For many teens who suspect they have depression, the first step is typically a trip to a primary care doctor's office. Primary care doctors can recognize and diagnose depression and give patients advice on next steps for treatment. Research shows that only relying on the primary care doctor is not as successful as working with a mental health professional. Often, primary care doctors refer the patient to a psychologist, psychiatrist, or clinical social worker.

Diagnosing depression involves conversations, screening, and tests. Doctors may talk to depressed teens about how they're feeling and try to get a sense of their symptoms. Depression screenings are questionnaires designed to look for the presence of depression symptoms and figure out how serious they are. One common questionnaire, the Patient Health Questionnaire, or PHQ-9, has nine questions. One question asks if the patient has "trouble concentrating on things, such as reading the newspaper or watching television."[11] Patients can answer that they've experienced the symptom "not at all," for "several days," for "more than half the days," or "nearly every day" over the past two weeks.

A primary care doctor can also run tests to rule out other explanations for the patient's symptoms. Hypothyroidism, for example, is a physical disorder that causes many of the same symptoms as depression. Treatments for depression and hypothyroidism are very different, however, and overlooking potential medical causes can have harmful effects.

WHAT ARE THE RISK FACTORS FOR TEEN DEPRESSION?

According to a 2017 study by the National Institute of Mental Health (NIMH), 13.3 percent of US residents ages twelve to seventeen had an episode of depression. This is a significant increase from 2005, when teen depression rates were at

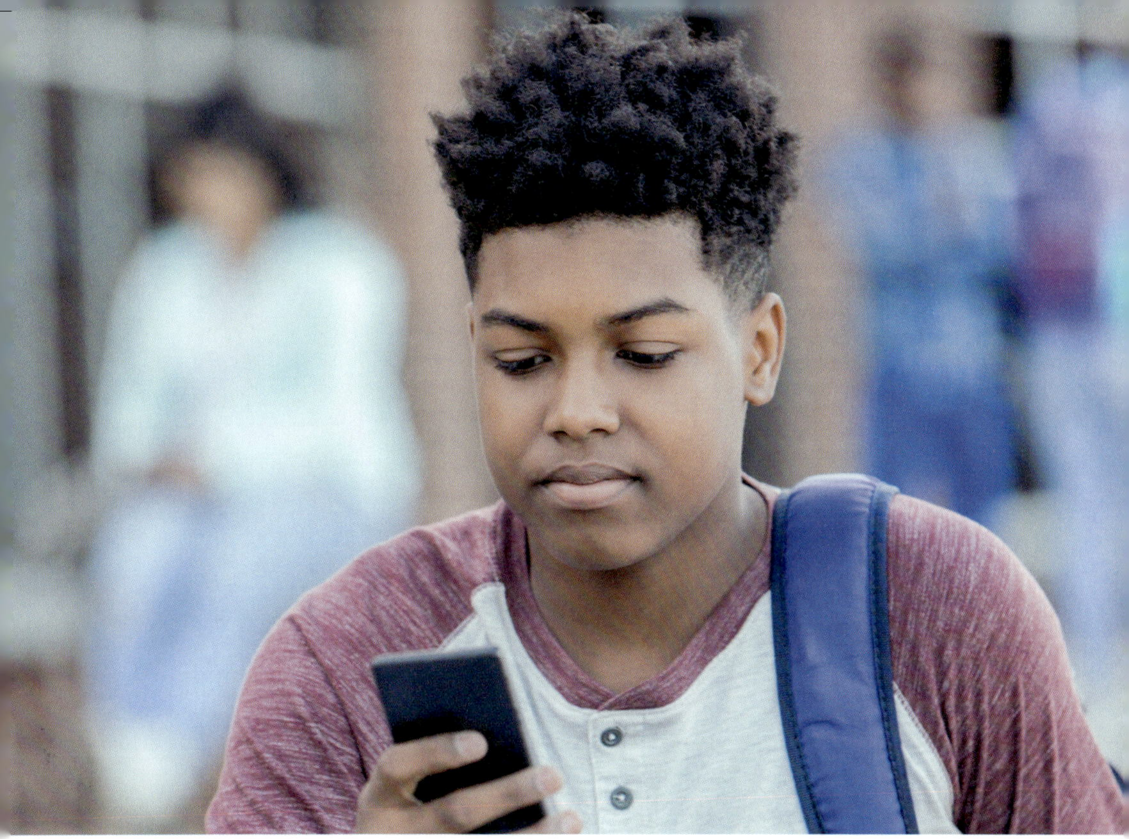

Studies have shown that social media use can cause low self-esteem. Low self-esteem is linked with depression.

8.7 percent. Experts are not sure why depression rates in teens have risen so sharply in just over a decade. The increase may be due to a greater ability and willingness from mental health professionals to diagnose depression in teens. Other studies pointed to teens' access to technology and social media, which can have negative effects on self-esteem. Technology may have also contributed to teens feeling a lack of community. But not all teens are equally likely to have a depressive episode. There are risk factors that increase a teen's probability of becoming depressed. A risk factor is a characteristic of a person or a factor in their environment that increases vulnerability to

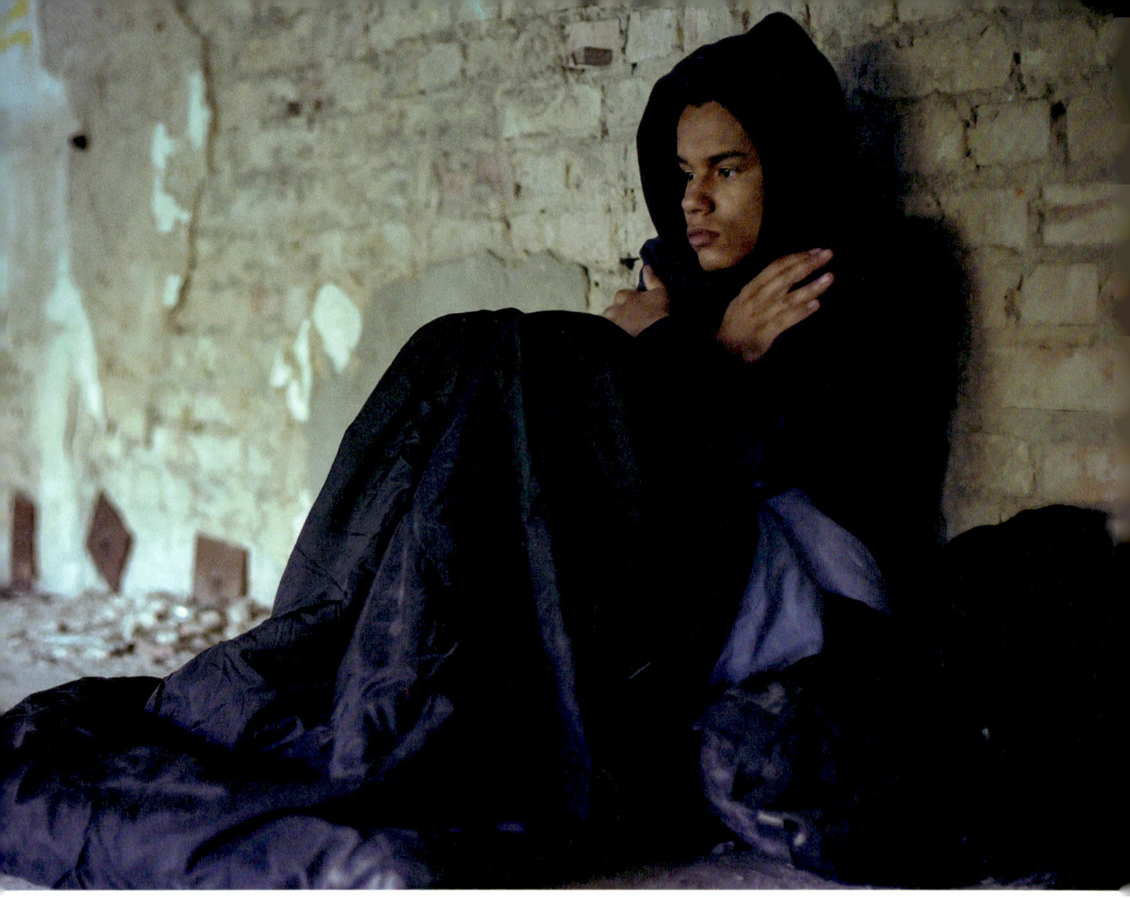

Environmental factors affect someone's likelihood of developing depression. For example, youths who live in poverty are at a higher risk.

an illness. Gender is a major risk factor for depression. Women and teen girls are much more likely than men and teen boys to be diagnosed with depression. No one is sure why this is the case. Before puberty, girls and boys get depressed at similar rates. Some researchers suggest, therefore, that the difference in depression rates is related to hormones. Others point to the discrimination women and girls face in society, suggesting that experiences of gender-based inequality may lead to depression.

Risk factors for depression can also be genetic or biological. Research into the experiences of identical twins suggests that some people are born more likely to become depressed, regardless of their life experiences. Since 1978, researchers have worked to identify whether there is a particular gene or set of genes that causes depression. So far, they have not been able to find a specific "depression gene." Instead, as an article in *Frontiers in Psychiatry* explains, "It is likely that the predisposition to [depressive disorders] is determined by the coordinated action of many genes and their interaction with each other and with diverse environmental factors."[12] In other words, many genes working together in combination with a person's surroundings and upbringing help cause depression. Researchers have also found that rates of depression are six times higher in youth who have depressed mothers. While this may be due to heredity, it can also be considered an environmental factor.

Environmental risk factors for depression include the circumstances in which a teen grows up and whether the teen experiences trauma or physical, emotional, or sexual abuse at a young age. People who live in poverty, for example, may go through severely stressful experiences like lacking secure access to food or housing and worrying about their physical safety. Over time, this stress takes its toll on the health of the body and brain. There is evidence that children who grow up in poverty are at a higher risk of developing depression. Children who are abused or neglected by their parents are at a higher risk of developing depression, as well.

Experiences of bullying, violence, racial and sexual discrimination, and exclusion often start in childhood. Exclusion can increase the likelihood of a depressive episode. For example, the hurdles that many LGBTQ teens face make them more vulnerable to depression and other mental disorders. The acronym LGBTQ stands for lesbian, gay, bisexual, transgender, and queer or questioning. The word *queer* is an umbrella term for people who do not identify as straight. LGBTQ people in general are two times more likely than heterosexual people to have a mental disorder, and teens who are bullied for being LGBTQ are more likely to become depressed. When Bree Leahy realized she was gay at age thirteen, she knew she would be treated badly by her classmates. “When I was at school, I was always the butt of the gay jokes and it made me feel ill,” the London native said in a radio interview.[13] The bullying she went through contributed to her depression.

DEPRESSION'S LINK TO OTHER ILLNESSES AND DISORDERS

Depressed teens are more likely than the general population to suffer from certain illnesses and disorders. For example, it’s very common for depressed people, including depressed teens, to suffer from anxiety disorders. Anxiety is excessive worry or fear about the future. People with anxiety disorders suffer from anxiety so intense it makes daily life difficult. About 60 percent of depressed people also suffer from symptoms of anxiety.

DSM-5'S EIGHT DEPRESSIVE DISORDERS

DEPRESSIVE DISORDER	CHARACTERISTICS
Disruptive Mood Dysregulation Disorder	Occurs in childhood, extreme bursts of anger
Major Depressive Disorder	Extended feelings of sadness, loss of motivation with daily activities
Persistent Depressive Disorder	Long-term depression, feelings of hopelessness and low self-esteem
Premenstrual Dysphoric Disorder	Occurs seven to ten days before period, extreme mood shifts and anxiety
Substance/Medication-Induced Depressive Disorder	Use of alcohol, drugs, or medication leads to depression
Depressive Disorder Due to Another Medical Condition	Depression linked to conditions such as AIDS, cancer, chronic back pain, and more
Other Specified Depressive Disorder	Doesn't fit into category of other depressive disorders, but still causes extreme distress; health care professional gives reason it doesn't fit in category
Unspecified Depressive Disorder	Doesn't fit into category of other depressive disorders, but still causes extreme distress; health care professional does not give reason it doesn't fit in category

The same is true for people with anxiety suffering symptoms of depression. Mental health professionals aren't sure why anxiety and depression go together so often. But they know anxiety disorders and depressive disorders can intensify each other, making the symptoms of both stronger. For Faith-Ann Bishop, the burden of both anxiety's and depression's painful feelings was overwhelming. She began self-harming in eighth grade. Going through the motions of daily life "was like asking me to climb Mount Everest in high heels," she told *Time* magazine.[14]

Youth with severe medical conditions such as cancer and irritable bowel syndrome (IBS) are more likely to experience depression. Young people with autism are also significantly more likely than non-autistic people to suffer from depression. Autism is a chronic condition that affects behavior, communication,

BIPOLAR DISORDER

Bipolar disorder is a mental illness with some similarities to depression. It used to be called manic depression or manic depressive disorder. People with bipolar disorder suffer depressive episodes, where they experience the symptoms of major depression. However, they also suffer from manic episodes, where they feel increased energy and elevated mood. During manic episodes, people with bipolar disorder may feel intense excitement and experience bursts of creativity and focus. However, manic episodes can also be scary and overwhelming, as sufferers may feel that their actions are beyond their control. Although depression and bipolar disorder are similar in some ways, the treatments for each disorder are different. Like teens suffering from depressive symptoms, teens who suspect they may be bipolar can talk with a doctor or health care professional.

and social skills. Like the relationship between depression and anxiety, the reasons behind the co-occurrence of these disorders are not completely understood and may be very complex. For example, people with physical illnesses like heart disease may be more likely to become depressed because of the stress and limitations of their illness. But it may also be true that depression negatively affects sufferers' physical health, so they are more likely to get sick. Or it could be that both explanations are partially true and that the disorders are related in a variety of ways.

SEASONAL AFFECTIVE DISORDER [SAD]

Seasonal Affective Disorder, often known as SAD, is a type of depressive disorder. People with SAD get symptoms of depression during particular seasons, usually during the winter months. The lower light and colder weather of the winter months can have a depressing effect on many people's moods. People who live where the lack of winter sunlight and colder temperatures are more dramatic are more likely to suffer from SAD. Younger people also have an increased risk. One of the most common treatments for SAD is light therapy. SAD sufferers can use a bright lamp called a light therapy box to get extra light during the day. People who suffer from non-seasonal depression can use these lamps as well. Other research has found a link between a lack of Vitamin D and SAD symptoms. Vitamin D may play an important role in helping to control mood.

CHAPTER
TWO

HOW DOES DEPRESSION AFFECT TEENS?

In the United States, depression is more common among teenagers than ever before. A 2019 study published in the *Journal of Abnormal Psychology* found that rates of teen depression had increased more than 52 percent in twelve years. Depression is a mental illness, but its effects go far beyond the mind to touch on every aspect of a teenager's life. Depression doesn't just cause sadness or invade the brain with unwelcome thoughts—it radiates throughout the body and steals much-needed energy. Depression makes teenagers more vulnerable to self-harming behaviors such as substance abuse and disordered eating, where people find themselves in harmful eating patterns such as eating too few calories or overeating. These and other risky behaviors caused by depression can be fatal.

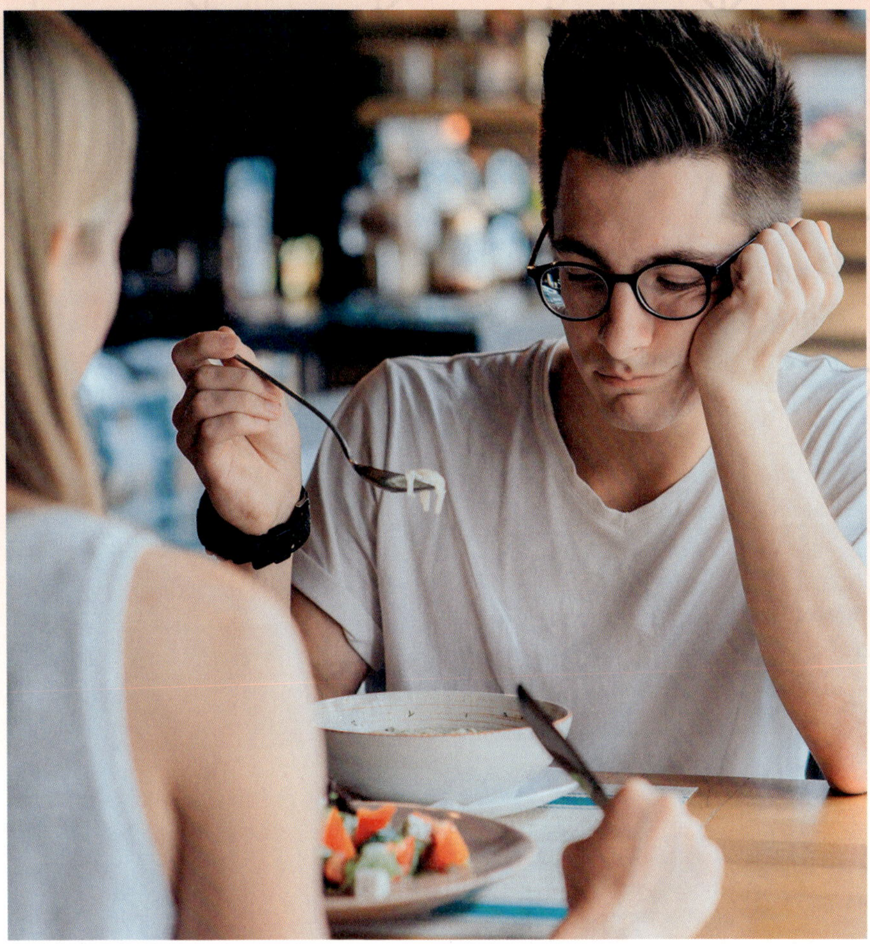

Depression affects a sufferer's physical health. For example, it can change a person's appetite or diet.

HOW IT FEELS TO BE DEPRESSED

Morgan Parker is a poet and YA author from California. In 2019, her novel *Who Put This Song On?* was published. The book is based on her own experiences as a depressed teen. At the beginning of the book, the narrator, also named Morgan, writes in her diary about her summer: "Summer is gone. I've spent it fighting with everyone around me and crying in bed all day. I'm so pathetic. I keep thinking, I wish I didn't do this. But it's like I can't help it. Because of my depression."[15]

Morgan puts a voice to the experiences of a lot of depressed teens. Depressed people may find themselves crying uncontrollably or every day. But depression can also show up as irritability, such as being constantly annoyed or unable to handle other people. This is especially true of teens, who are more likely to show anger than both older and younger depressed people. Morgan spends her summer "fighting with everyone around [her]."

Brynn, who did not give her last name, had a similar experience with her family. She became depressed and started fighting with her parents. "My siblings, whom I used to be so close with, now asked me 'where the old Brynn was' when I snapped at them," Brynn remembers.[16] Fighting with loved ones can feel terrible—depressed teens may feel guilty for venting their anger and isolate themselves. Without treatment, the sadness and anger of depression remain, making relationships with others more difficult.

> **"My siblings, whom I used to be so close with, now asked me 'where the old Brynn was' when I snapped at them."[16]**
>
> ***—Brynn, teen with depression***

When they're not sad and angry, some depressed teens may feel a sense of numbness or emptiness. It's common for depressed teens to lose motivation and become uninterested in things they used to find important or fun. Comedian Patti Harrison remembers what it was like to be depressed in the first few years of college. She started cutting classes and didn't want to go out or participate in activities. She felt sadness and anger as well as a sense of pointlessness and emptiness. "How I experience depression was like, at first there was crying," Harrison told interviewer John Moe. "But then . . . there was a long time where it was just kind of like feeling indifferent. . . . Everything sucks, everyone's bad, there's nothing of any worth here."[17] Harrison eventually left college without getting a degree.

> **"Everything sucks, everyone's bad, there's nothing of any worth here."[17]**
>
> ***—Patti Harrison, comedian***

Harrison's academic struggles are common for depressed teens. According to a 2005 study published in the *Journal of Mental Health Policy and Economics*, having clinical depression was associated with a GPA decrease of .49, or half a letter grade. This link between depression and performance extends past school into all areas of life. According to the World Health Organization, depression is the number one cause of disability throughout the world. More than any other illness, depression lowers the sufferers' ability to work and function fully in public and daily life. Depression takes a toll on the body. It can show itself in the form of muscle tension, headaches, and other types of chronic pain. It can also be an exhausting illness. Another common symptom of depression among teens is sleep disturbance. Sleep is especially important for teens. According to the National Sleep Foundation, teens need an average of eight to ten hours of sleep a night, which is more than the average adult. Getting enough sleep can help teens manage their stress and emotions. In contrast, sleep disturbances worsen other symptoms of depression, like irritability and an inability to concentrate. This is an example of the vicious cycle of depression. Depression makes it difficult for sufferers to take care of themselves in simple ways, such as showering, eating well, and exercising. In turn, this lack of care deepens depression symptoms and produces shame and guilt, making it even more difficult to reach out for help.

In rare cases, depressed teens may also suffer from psychosis. Psychosis is an inability to tell the difference between real life and delusions or hallucinations. Delusions are false beliefs, and hallucinations are sensory experiences of things that are not really there. A depressed teen suffering from delusions might, for example, believe they have committed a murder that they did not really commit. The guilt and shame of this imaginary murder would feel very real and overwhelming.

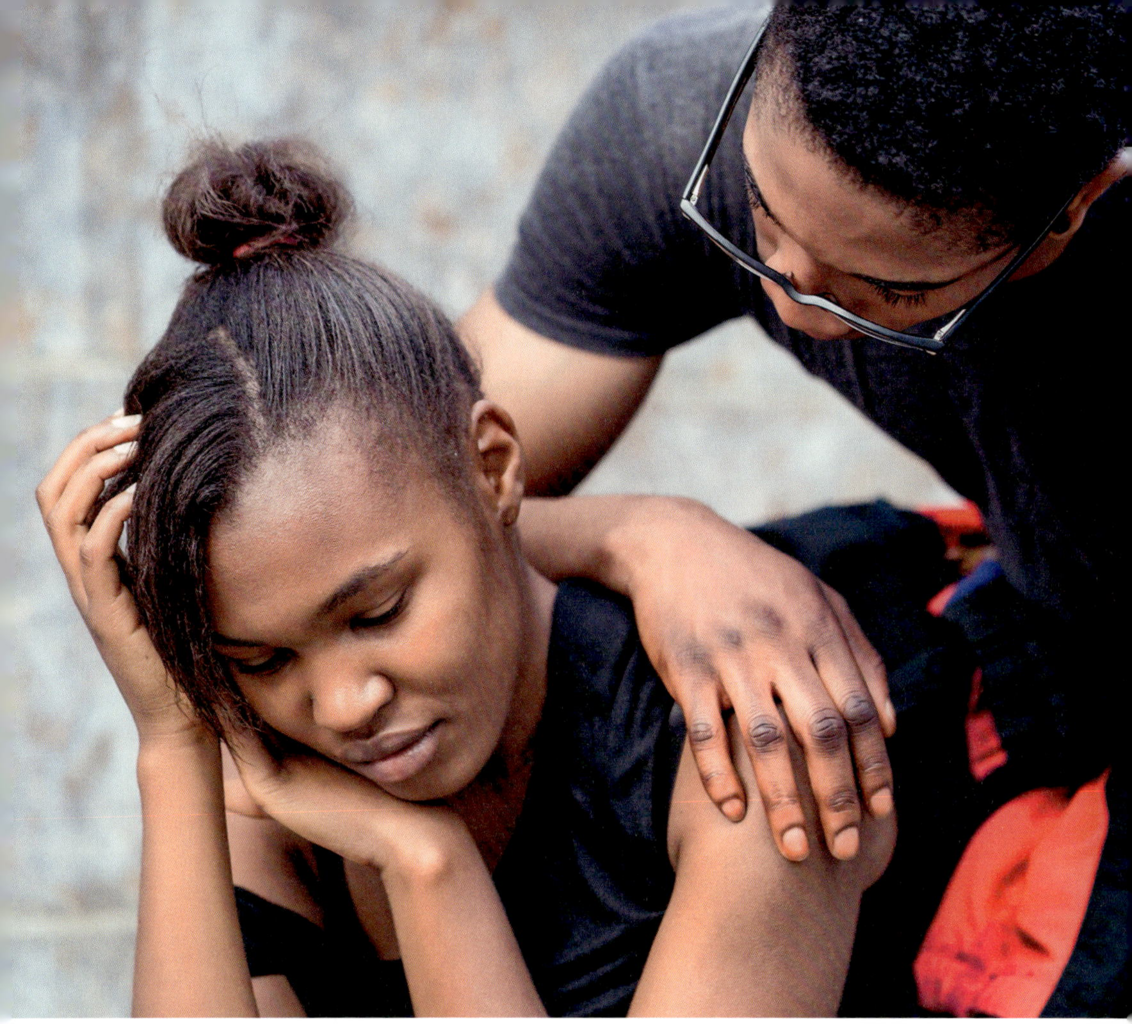

Depression can put a strain on relationships. People with depression may isolate themselves.

DEPRESSION AND RELATIONSHIPS

Depression makes it more difficult for teens to build and maintain strong relationships. The mood disruptions of depression can make family relationships more difficult. In the wider world, depressed teens may struggle with poor self-esteem, which results in negative self-talk that makes them believe that they are not loved or accepted by others.

Model and actress Cara Delevingne has spoken about the severe depression she went through as a teen. Delevingne lived a peaceful, privileged life, but she struggled to fit in with her peers. She was bullied, and she blamed herself for her low self-esteem and loneliness. "I felt alienated and alone, because I was like, what's wrong with me?" Delevingne remembers. "I always wanted people to love me, so I never got angry with them; I turned my anger on to myself."[18] Delevingne left school at age fifteen partly because of her depression.

The ups and downs of dating and relationships can be very difficult for depressed teens. A study published in 2011 in the *Journal of Clinical Child and Adolescent Psychology* found that problem-solving in relationships was more difficult for depressed teens. In other words, it may be more difficult for teens with depression to manage conflict with others and negotiate long-lasting relationships. And according to research published in *Behavioral Sciences,* negative relationship experiences like a breakup or a negative sexual experience increase suicide risk in teens. For Erika Wenzel, a breakup during her junior year of high school triggered an episode of depression. She went from mourning her relationship to feeling painful self-hatred and sadness. Her depression damaged her relationship with her friends, and she started avoiding school and her family. "No one seemed to understand it wasn't about a breakup

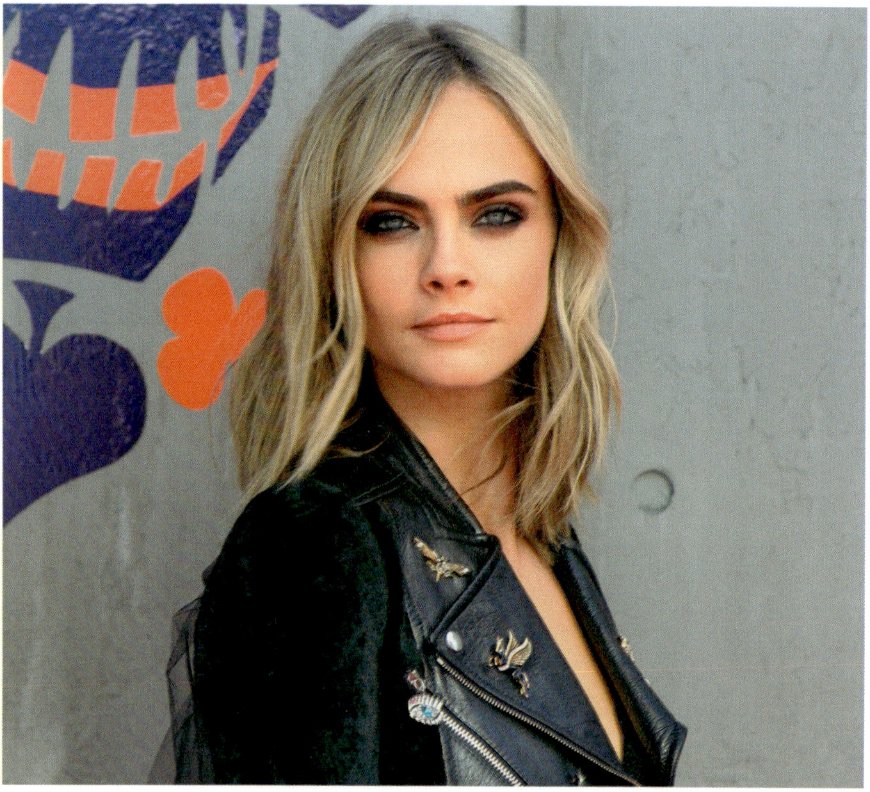

Many celebrities have spoken out about mental health. Actress and model Cara Delevingne had depression during her teen years.

anymore," Wenzel writes about that time. "My depression was all-consuming, with no single cause."[19]

People with depression often long for emotional support and connection, but they feel unable to seek it out because of their symptoms. This contradiction is part of depression's vicious cycle: depression makes people isolate themselves, and that loneliness and isolation ends up worsening the effects of depression.

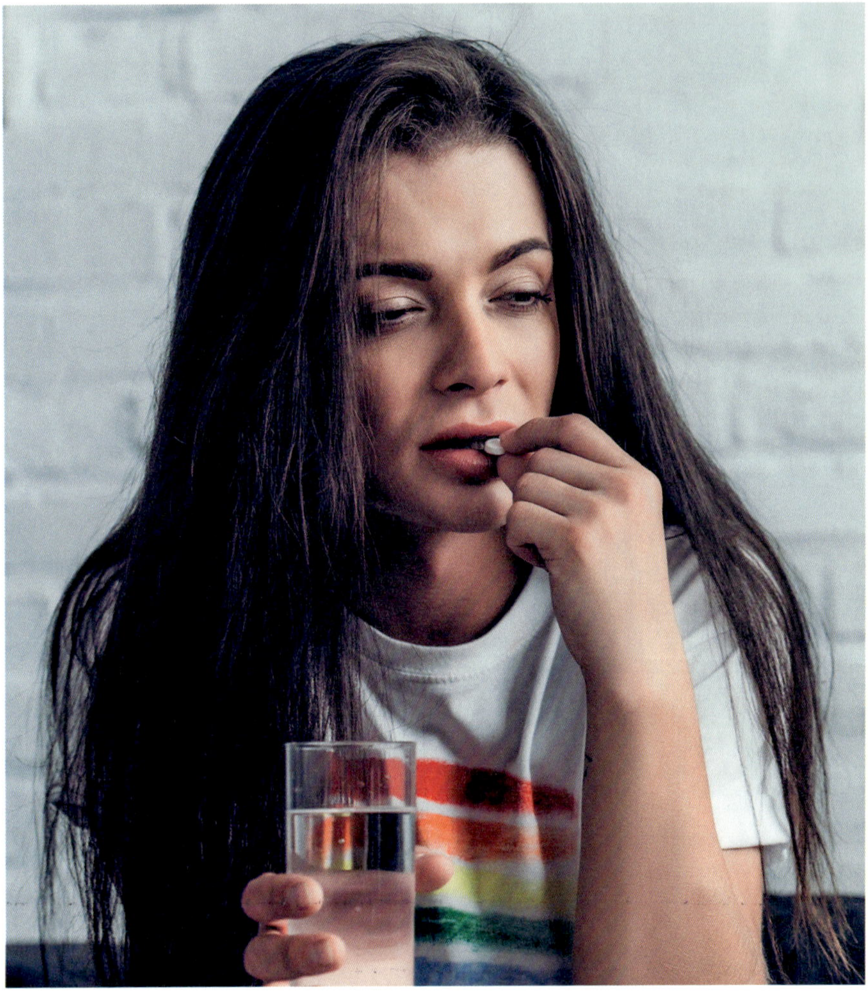

People who are depressed may use drugs or alcohol to try to make themselves feel better. This can worsen their depression.

DEPRESSION AND HARMFUL BEHAVIORS

Depression is associated with substance abuse, as well as physical self-harm and disordered eating. The connections between these disorders are complex. In some cases, depressed teens turn to substances or self-harm in order to cope with the unbearable feelings depression produces. In others, teens who abuse substances or develop eating disorders may also find themselves becoming depressed as the effects of their disorders cause suffering and isolation. Sometimes, the cause-and-effect relationship between depression and other harmful behaviors is unclear and complex.

Depression's connection to alcohol and marijuana is one of these complicated relationships. According to the Addiction Center, about half of all teens who abuse substances also have a mental illness such as depression or anxiety. A 2014 study published in *Drug and Alcohol Dependence* surveyed ninth graders on mental illness symptoms, emotional health, and drug and alcohol use. The study found that students who reported more depressive symptoms were more likely to start using substances like alcohol and tobacco and continue for a long time. Depressant drugs like alcohol can create feelings of calmness and help lonely people ease their social anxiety. However, some of alcohol's effects, like loss of concentration and tiredness, overlap with the symptoms of depression. Alcohol and marijuana, the other primary drug abused by teens, have sedating effects. This can further maintain someone's depression. Other drugs, such as heroin, give people intense feelings of pleasure and excitement. This is an especially tempting effect for depressed people who struggle to feel any kind of enjoyment in life.

For Tracey Helton Mitchell, pain medication abuse became her self-medication for teen depression. Mitchell suffered from untreated depression from the age of twelve, and she started abusing the prescription painkiller Vicodin as a teen. Eventually, Mitchell became a heroin addict. "I would argue a lot of people start using opioids as antidepressants . . . then the solution becomes the problem," Mitchell told BuzzFeed News.[20]

> "I would argue a lot of people start using opioids as antidepressants . . . then the solution becomes the problem."[20]
>
> *—Tracey Helton Mitchell, person recovering from heroin addiction*

Binge-eating disorder is a condition where people overeat, sometimes to the point of sickness. People with binge-eating disorder do not feel control over their overeating sessions and feel shame and guilt after eating. Binge-eating disorder is strongly associated with depression, and many people with the disorder are also depressed. The link between depression and binge eating is especially strong for teen girls.

TEEN DEPRESSION AND SUICIDE

Depression can be a contributor to suicidal ideation. Suicide is the second-leading cause of death for US teens. It's impossible to know for sure how many suicide deaths are the result of depression. Some teens may suffer from illnesses or conditions other than depression and die by suicide. Others may die by suicide after suffering from undiagnosed depression. However, experts agree that depression is a major contributor to suicidal thoughts and behavior among teens. "I don't think it is an exaggeration at all to say that we have a mental health crisis among adolescents in the US," said Jean Twenge, a psychologist who studies teen mental health.[21] Teens who have survived suicide attempts often remember how ending their own lives seemed at one time to be the only solution to their pain. They did not actually want to die, but they felt trapped by pain and wanted it to end.

> **"I don't think it is an exaggeration at all to say that we have a mental health crisis among adolescents in the US."[21]**
>
> ***—Jean Twenge, psychologist and mental health researcher***

Some teens are at especially high risk of suicide. According to the Emergency Taskforce on Black Youth Suicide and Mental Health, black children under the age of thirteen were twice as likely to die by suicide than white children in 2019. One survey found that many black teens have experienced traumatic online racial images and videos. Other research pointed to the role of trauma in black communities, such as discrimination, economic insecurity, and neighborhood violence.

Teen boys in general are about three times more likely than teen girls to die by suicide. However, teen girls contemplate suicide more than teen boys. In 2017, when teen suicides were at an all-time high in the United States, teens in rural areas were 80 percent more likely to die by suicide than teens in large cities. Much of that increase was due to significantly higher rates of suicide among older teenage boys. Experts believe that the increase in suicides in rural areas of the United States is linked to the effects of the opioid epidemic, or a widespread abuse of opioid drugs. LGBTQ teens

TEEN DEPRESSION IN MEDIA AND ENTERTAINMENT

TV shows such as *Euphoria* on HBO and *13 Reasons Why* on Netflix feature teen characters who suffer from depression. Some of these shows draw on the real-life experiences of their creators and their memories of being depressed teens. Sam Levinson, who adapted *Euphoria* from an Israeli miniseries, struggled with substance abuse and depression for years. However, these series have also faced criticism for promoting myths about teens and depression. For example, the first season of the TV show *13 Reasons Why* is about a teenage girl named Hannah who dies by suicide. She leaves cassette tapes with messages for friends and family after her death, explaining her pain. Some of *13 Reasons Why*'s writers have personal experience with mental illness. However, critics pointed out that the show might make suicide seem like a glamorous choice instead of a tragic one. It could send the message that suicide is a way of sending messages to others, instead of a choice that ends communication forever. This, in turn, can cause suicide contagion. Suicide contagion is the direct and indirect exposure of suicide increasing the likelihood of someone dying by suicide.

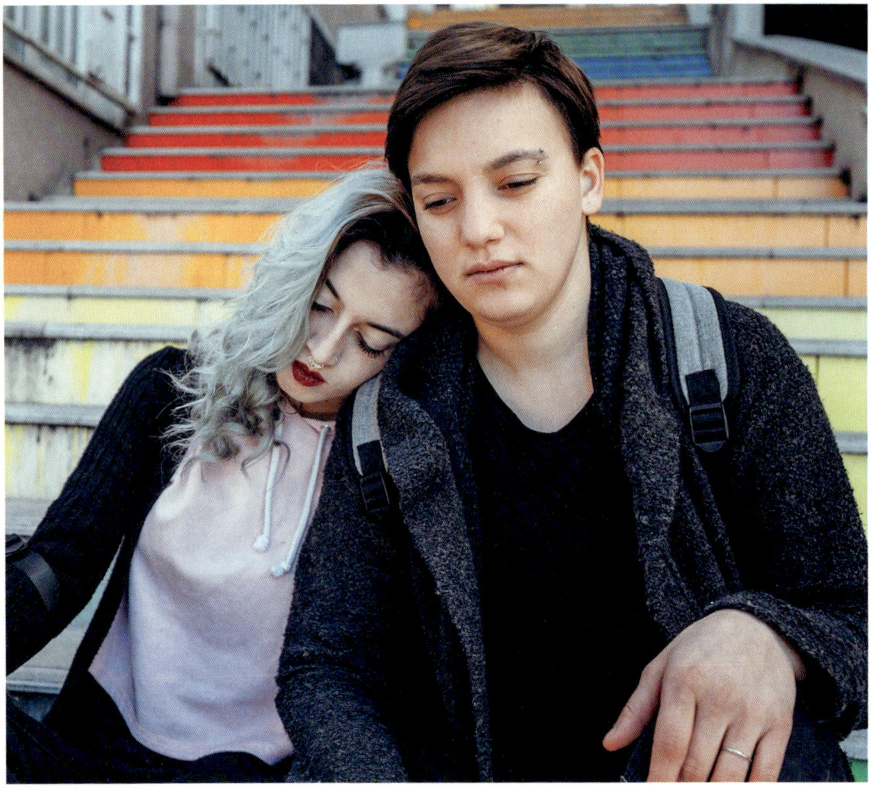

LGBTQ teens are more likely than straight teens to attempt suicide. Many feel shamed by society.

are more likely to consider or attempt suicide than straight teens are. Attempted suicide rates are especially high among young transgender people. In 2018, 51 percent of transgender teen males, 42 percent of teens who identified as neither male nor female, and 30 percent of transgender teen females reported attempting suicide. Patti Harrison was not yet out as a transgender woman when she attempted suicide in her late teens. She was suffering from a deep depression and remembers feeling that "it was so shameful to be trans."[22] She saw a suicide attempt as a way to demonstrate the pain she was

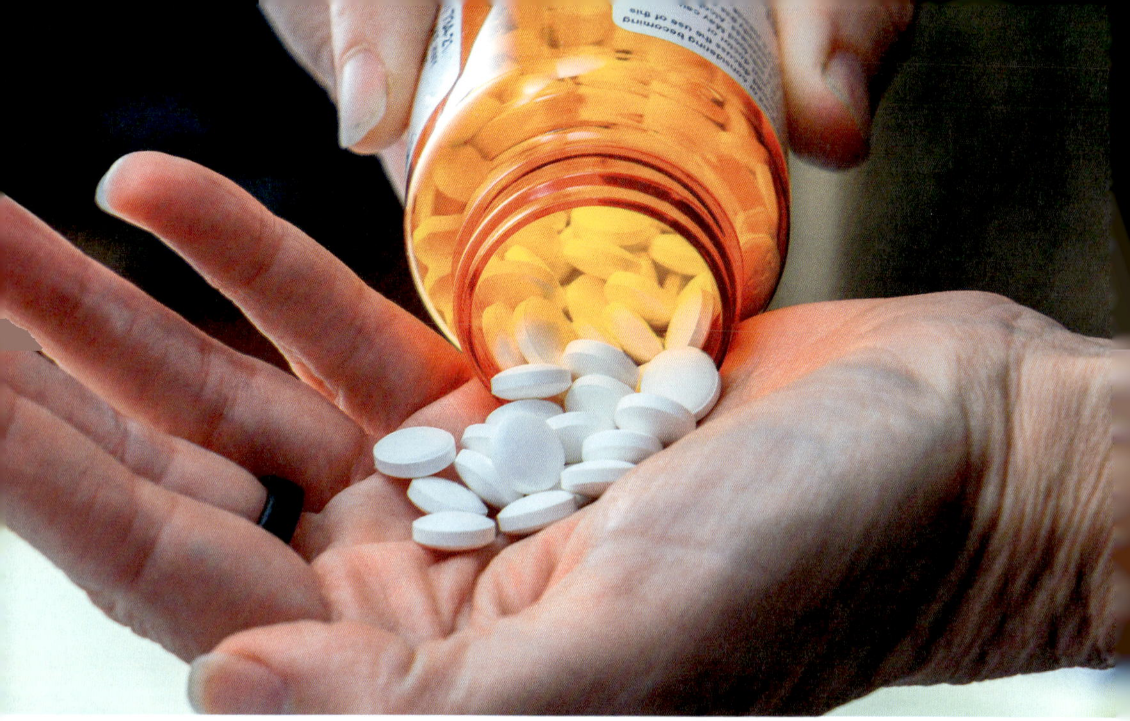

In 2017, the opioid epidemic was declared a public health emergency. Many overdoses have occurred since the start of the crisis in the 1990s.

feeling, a state of mind she now feels was her depression telling her lies. After her attempt, Harrison realized immediately that she wanted to live and was able to help herself.

The sharp increase in suicide among teens may not capture the full story of teens and suicidal behavior. Some teens die from accidents or overdoses that may or may not be the result of suicidal thoughts. The opioid epidemic in the United States has claimed many thousands of lives. People who frequently use opioids such as fentanyl or heroin are at a high risk of overdose. Overdosing occurs when someone takes more of a drug than the body can handle, which can lead to death. In many cases, fatal overdoses happen accidentally. However, some people may take higher and higher doses of drugs as a way of attempting suicide. They may also use drugs heavily without caring whether they live or die, a sort of "gray area" between suicide and accidental overdose. In 2017, doctors Mark Gold and Benjamin Srivastava reviewed information on opioid overdose deaths in the United States. They estimated that around 14 percent of teen opioid overdose deaths were probably suicides. The doctors recommended that patients who overdose on drugs receive mental health screenings and care.

TEENS AND DEPRESSION WORLDWIDE

About 15 percent of people in high-income countries will suffer from depression at some point in their lives. Depression rates tend to be higher in wealthier countries. One possible reason this is true is that wealthy countries tend to have large income gaps between richer and poorer people, and the experience of inequality can lead to depression. According to the World Health Organization, rates of depression are especially high in India, where a 2016 study found that about 20 percent of teens suffer from some type of mental illness. In India, suicide is the leading cause of death for people age thirteen to seventeen. Teenagers in India face common stressors and challenges such as problems at school, trouble within families, and emotional isolation. Like teens in the United States, many depressed teens in India aren't sure where to go for support. A 2016 survey found that almost a third of Indian teens with mental health problems did not talk to anyone else about their symptoms.

The National Suicide Prevention Lifeline is available around the clock to any person who has suicidal thoughts or urges. The phone number is 1-800-273-8255, and live chat services are available at any time at https://suicidepreventionlifeline.org/chat/.

CHAPTER THREE

HOW DOES TEEN DEPRESSION AFFECT SOCIETY?

When a teenager suffers from depression, the community suffers too. Depression robs teens of access to their energy and talents, and it isolates them from the people who care about them. It delays them from reaching their full potential and makes it more difficult to grow and share with others. Many depressed teens suffer in silence. A lack of information about mental illness and the fear of negative stigma, or judgment, mean that many teens stay depressed even when treatment is available.

WHEN A LOVED ONE IS DEPRESSED

It's painful to watch a loved one suffer from depression. The family and friends of depressed teens may not know how

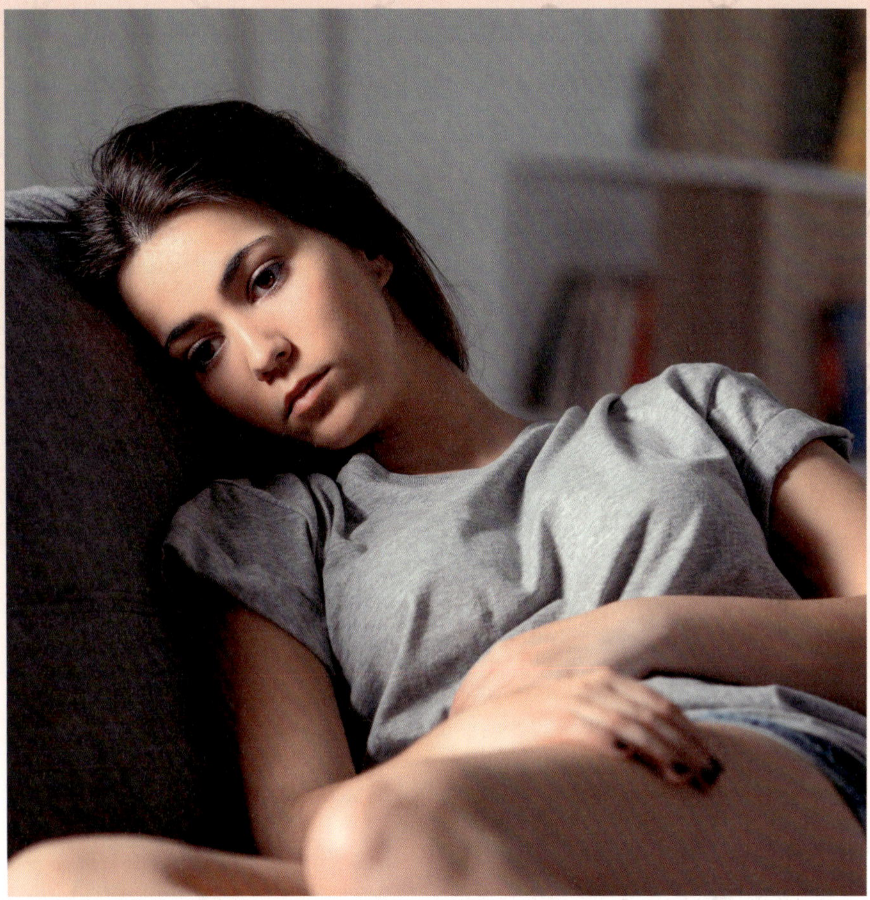

Depressed teens may feel a lack of motivation or self-confidence. This can stop them from reaching their full potential.

to help, or even reach, a depressed loved one. In 2017, an anonymous woman wrote for the *Guardian* about her memories of her sister in the depths of her depression. "You slept all afternoon and night," the woman wrote. "I would lay my cardigan over you so you wouldn't get cold. But I don't think it made a difference. You were lost to us, floating in some different universe with no anchor or thread holding you to us."[23] This woman's sense of distance and alienation from her sister echoed the isolation that depressed people feel. Depressed teens can feel cut off from other people, and their loved ones can feel cut off from them. Friends of depressed teens may struggle to understand why their friend is withdrawn or always seems sad and angry. Nicola Morgan, a youth counselor, describes having a depressed friend this way: "Being a good friend in that situation can be frightening, frustrating and worrying and it can make you feel powerless. You sense that it's important not to say the wrong thing but sometimes *everything* seems like the wrong thing."[24] This is another example of depression's vicious cycle. Depressed teens need the understanding and support of their loved ones, but depression makes that understanding and support difficult to offer and to receive.

"Being a good friend in that situation can be frightening, frustrating and worrying and it can make you feel powerless. You sense that it's important not to say the wrong thing but sometimes *everything* seems like the wrong thing."[24]

—Nicola Morgan, youth counselor

Losing a loved one as a result of depression is a devastating experience. When depression claims the life of teenagers, their friends and family are left with lifelong grief. People who lose a loved one to suicide are at increased risk of depression and suicide attempts themselves. Shellie and Jeff Sterner from Pennsylvania lost their son Joshua to suicide when he was nineteen years old. Joshua's sister Erin was twenty-two years old at the time. Joshua also left behind two young daughters. Joshua's parents and sister went to counseling in the wake of his death. Joshua's mother volunteered for a time as a grief counselor, and Joshua's father speaks publicly about how his life changed after his son's death. But the pain of his death has never gone away: "Everything that was normal was ripped away," Erin told a reporter. "The sibling I was the closest to . . . wasn't there."[25]

DEPRESSED PARENTS

When people with untreated depression become parents, their depression affects the way they raise their children. Megan Smith, PhD, studies depression in parents and its effects. Smith has found that a parent's depression can have a strong negative impact on their children. According to Smith, depressed parents are less likely to respond to their children's emotions. They may be more likely to neglect parenting tasks, such as taking their children to doctor's appointments. Depression also "disrupts a parent's ability to . . . participate in the community," Smith says. In other words, depressed parents, like depressed teens, are more likely to be socially isolated. As a result, the children of depressed parents are more likely to suffer from health and behavior problems. They are more vulnerable to symptoms and risk factors of depression, such as low self-worth and a tendency to blame themselves.

Quoted in "Parental Depression: How It Affects a Child," Yale Medicine, *n.d. www.yalemedicine.org.*

DEPRESSION IS A THIEF

Depression steals the time and energy of its sufferers. Depressive episodes can last for months or years, especially if they are not treated. People with depression miss out on time to connect with others and grow into their true selves. The teen years are a crucial time to discover passions and lay the

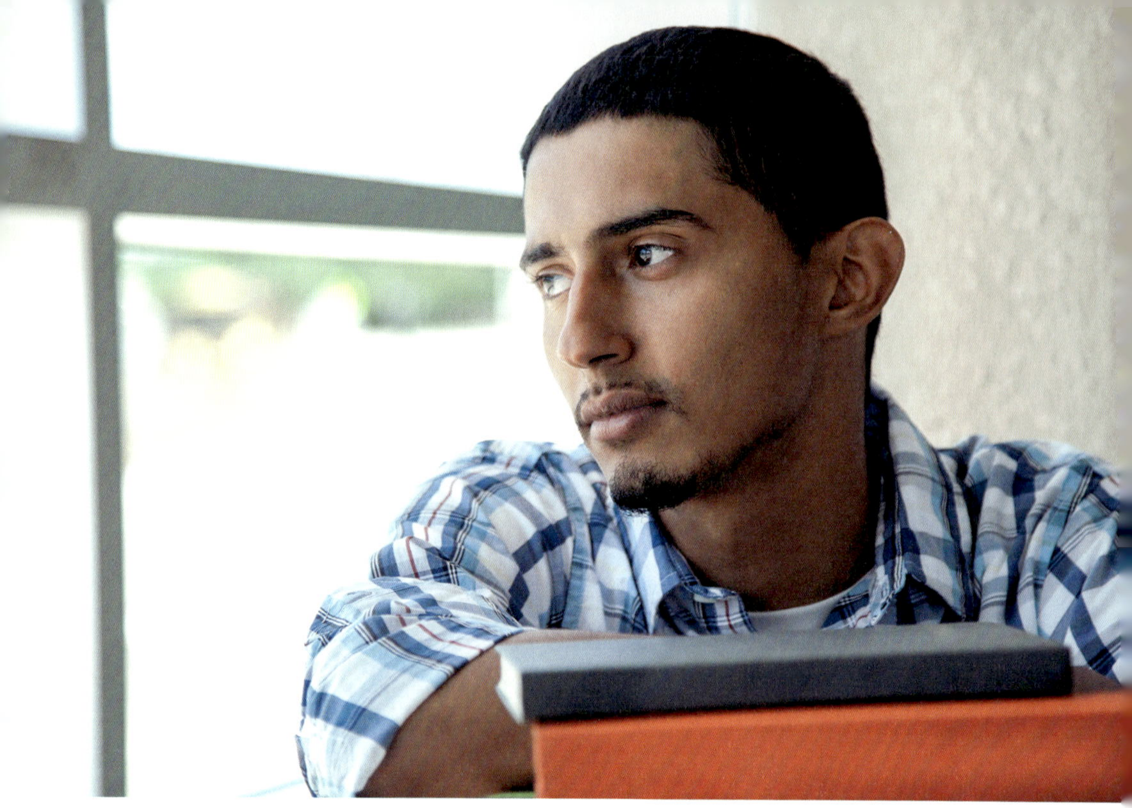

Depression can lower a teen's motivation to go to school or participate in activities. This may further isolate someone.

groundwork for a full, satisfying adult life. Depression can cause teens to underachieve in school and at work. And the feelings of hopelessness and worthlessness that depression creates can make preparing for the future seem pointless. Many adults who suffered from depression as teens live with regret as adults. As adults, they may suffer from imposter syndrome, or feelings of inadequacy that don't go away, even when they succeed. They may deprive themselves and others of their greatness.

Carl, a man in his midthirties, started suffering from depression in his midteens. "I struggled to focus on anything for any period of time, from work to going to the gym, or even just a shopping trip," Carl remembers.[26] Eventually, Carl lost a relationship with a man he loved because of his depression. In adulthood, Carl works hard to manage his symptoms with therapy, medication, and his own reading and research.

Robin Thompson grew up in her aunt's home in Brooklyn, New York. She started suffering from depression as a child, but she was not diagnosed until she was well into adulthood. She remembers the illness as disabling. "[Depression is] almost like someone has their hands around your neck," Thompson told the *New York Times*.[27] Thompson struggled in school, and in her teen years, she did not go to high school. She began misusing alcohol. For most of her adult life, Thompson was addicted to alcohol and neglectfully mothered three children. In her fifties, Thompson sought therapy for her illness. She stopped drinking and misusing drugs and began working toward a high school diploma. At age fifty-four, Thompson described herself as happier than she had ever been, even though her past is laced with pain and regret.

MENTAL ILLNESS AND INSTITUTIONALIZATION

Some depressed people, including depressed teens, go to hospitals during mental health crises. There are two types of hospitalization for depressed patients: voluntary and involuntary. In voluntary hospitalization, depressed patients decide they need

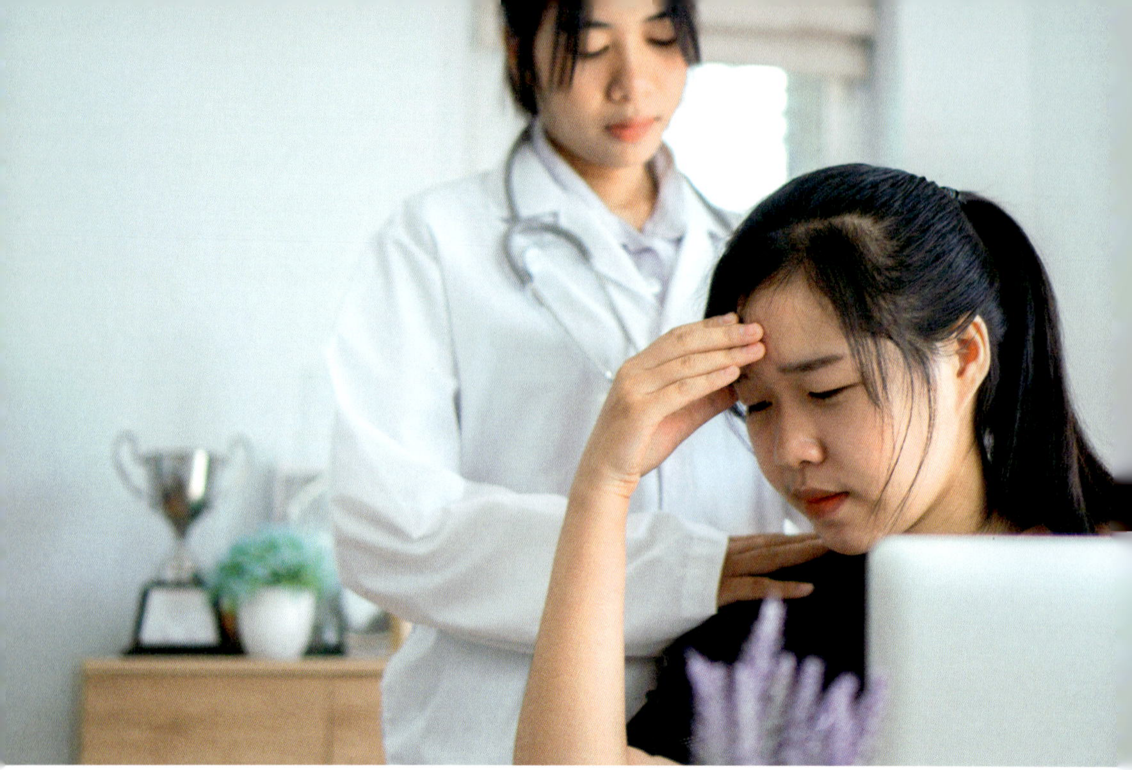

Depressed people who are considering suicide may need hospitalization. Hospitalization can be voluntary or involuntary.

full-time medical care because of an issue like suicidal ideation or because they want support for a challenge, such as adjusting to a new medication. Involuntary hospitalization occurs when medical professionals decide that a patient is in danger of harm to self or others and needs to be hospitalized immediately. The criteria for ordering an involuntary hospitalization vary from state to state. Involuntary hospitalizations typically only last a few days, and voluntary hospitalizations can last up to several months. However, staying for a few weeks is more common. There are special hospitals and parts of hospitals dedicated to treating people with mental illnesses. Less than 10 percent of depression cases require some period of hospitalization.

MENTAL ILLNESS AND STIGMA

Stigma is a feeling of shame or negative judgment that society attaches to some people, beliefs, actions, or conditions. Even though depression is very common, it is also highly stigmatized. People with depression face several negative stereotypes. Some people believe that those with depression are lazy, simply need to take better care of themselves, or just need to get over their anger and sadness. Depressed people can internalize these thoughts and begin to believe them. This stigma makes it more difficult for depressed teens to properly understand their own symptoms, to reach out to each other, and to embrace the need for treatment and support.

When Kevin Breel was a teenager, he suffered from severe depression. However, he felt an intense need to seem fine to his community. He put a lot of pressure on himself to succeed academically and keep up his popular, athletic image. He would walk into school and "smile, laugh, high-five people, and put on a total front," Breel remembers. After having suicidal thoughts, Breel reached out for help. But he was even more afraid of the judgment of others than he was of facing his own dark feelings. "We live in a world where if you break your arm, everyone runs over to

> "We live in a world where if you break your arm, everyone runs over to sign your cast, but if you tell people you're depressed, everyone runs the other way."[28]
>
> *—Kevin Breel, depressed teen*

sign your cast, but if you tell people you're depressed, everyone runs the other way," Breel told *Today*.[28] Breel eventually made a TED talk video encouraging others to talk about their depression. As of January 2020, it had almost a million YouTube views.

Seeking treatment for mental illness is often stigmatized as well. Teens who go to therapy or take medication may fear harsh judgment from others. According to psychiatrist Louisa Steinberg, "Stigmatization of mental health treatment . . . prevents those who need it from seeking out help."[29] Teens may be aware they are suffering from depression but not feel able to get the help they need. Untreated depression can have powerful and often unexpected effects in the lives of the depressed person and their families.

> **"Stigmatization of mental health treatment . . . prevents those who need it from seeking out help."[29]**
>
> ***—Louisa Steinberg, psychiatrist***

Prachi Gupta is a journalist from Pittsburgh, Pennsylvania. She and her brother Yush grew up in an Indian American home in a mostly white community in the 1990s. Gupta and her brother felt the isolation and discrimination of living in a mostly white area, which left them at greater risk of depression. In addition, Gupta's family and her culture discouraged talking about mental health issues.

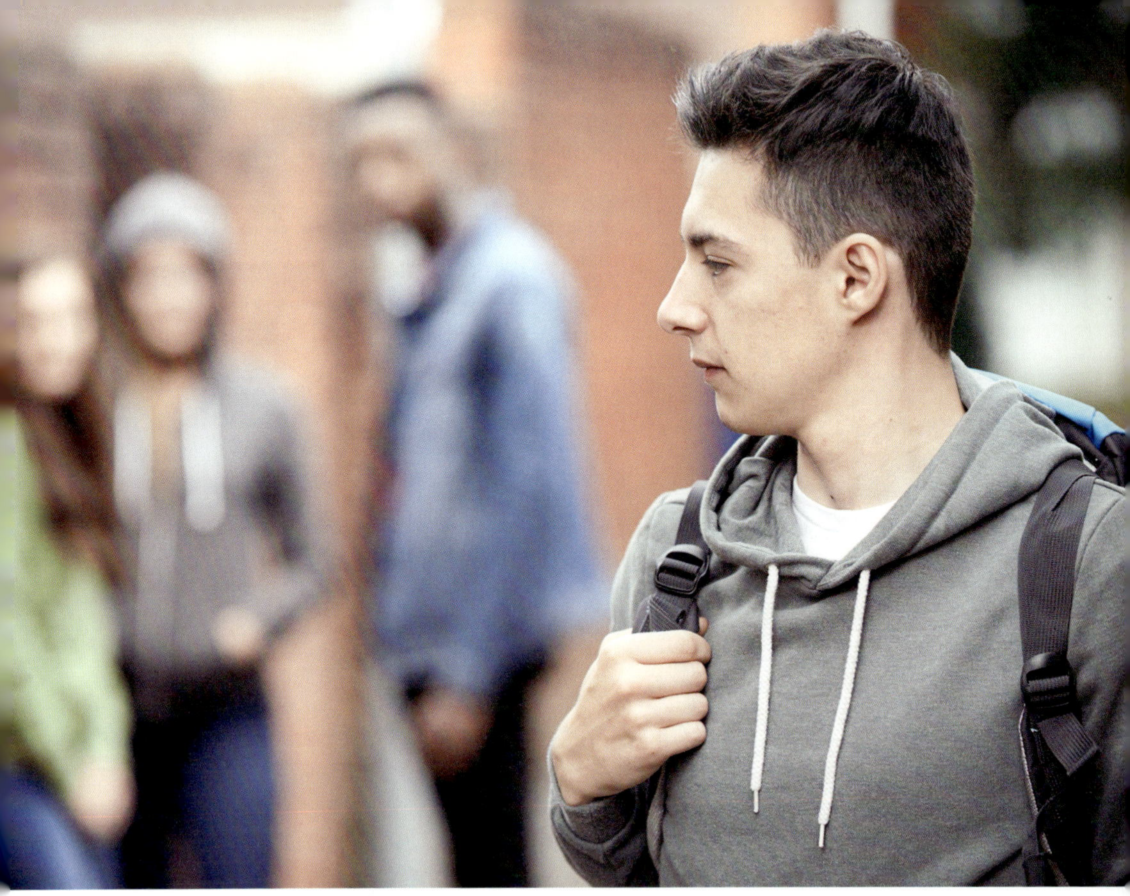

Someone who is depressed might not seek out help because of social or cultural stigma. Someone may feel judged for his or her mental illness.

Gupta points out that while minorities in the United States are more likely to have suicidal ideation, Asian Americans are less likely than any other racial group to seek therapy. This stigma against discussing or treating mental health issues is especially strong for men. Common gender roles, or expectations for men and women, encourage men and boys to appear strong and in control. In Gupta's family, men were not expected to express sadness, and seeking help with difficult feelings was perceived as weak.

SCHOOL COUNSELORS AND TEEN DEPRESSION

For teens in middle school and high school, school counselors can be a free resource for mental health information and advice. School counselors in the United States typically get master's degrees in and take courses in individual and group counseling. School counselors cannot diagnose mental illnesses such as depression. However, they can meet with students one-on-one and lead group sessions where students meet together to discuss their challenges and offer support. School counselors can also serve as a link between students and families. They can help students advocate for medical treatment with their parents and help them find resources outside of school. School counselors can also help depressed teens succeed in school and get the accommodations they need. Counselors are a huge help to students, but counselors are sometimes overstretched in schools. The number of school counselors in US schools is rising, but it's still low. As of 2019, there was an average of one school counselor for every 455 K–12 students in the United States. The American School Counselor Association recommends a much lower ratio of one counselor for every 250 students.

Yush Gupta was charming and a standout student. "It was apparent, from a young age, that Yush was brilliant," Prachi remembers.[30] When he got to college, however, Yush began suffering from depression that went untreated. In his early twenties, he attempted suicide. Gupta's family didn't discuss Yush's suicidal ideation. "None of us even told our tightknit extended family for months," Gupta writes, "perhaps over the fear of shame, or perhaps because of fear he, or we, would be seen differently."[31]

In adulthood, Prachi Gupta began seeing a therapist to work through her own mental health issues. Yush occasionally took antidepressants, or medication designed to ease his symptoms. However, he didn't share much about his mental illness with others. In his late twenties, Yush died. He underwent cosmetic surgery to lengthen his legs, a risky procedure he thought would make him look more masculine and gain him respect. He died suddenly from a complication after the surgery. Gupta believes that stigma against mental health treatment for men is partly to blame for her brother's death. "Once you get into a depressive state, it tells you a lot of lies," says Reka Prasad, Gupta's therapist.[32] Gupta believes that the lies depression told her brother, and the silence around his illness, led to him seeking the surgery that cost him his life. Like Yush, many others suffer from depression in silence because of their religious, racial, and ethnic communities.

CHAPTER FOUR

HOW CAN WE TREAT AND PREVENT TEEN DEPRESSION?

There are safe, effective treatments for teens who suffer from depression. Two supported treatments for adolescents are interpersonal psychotherapy (IPT) and cognitive behavioral therapy (CBT). While antidepressant medications may work for many depression sufferers, depressed teens can also go to therapy to learn to take good care of themselves in ways that help relieve symptoms of depression. Three key steps to treating teen depression are raising awareness of the disorder, ending the stigma against mental illness and treatment, and making health care easier for teens to access. There are people and programs working on all three fronts to treat and prevent teen depression.

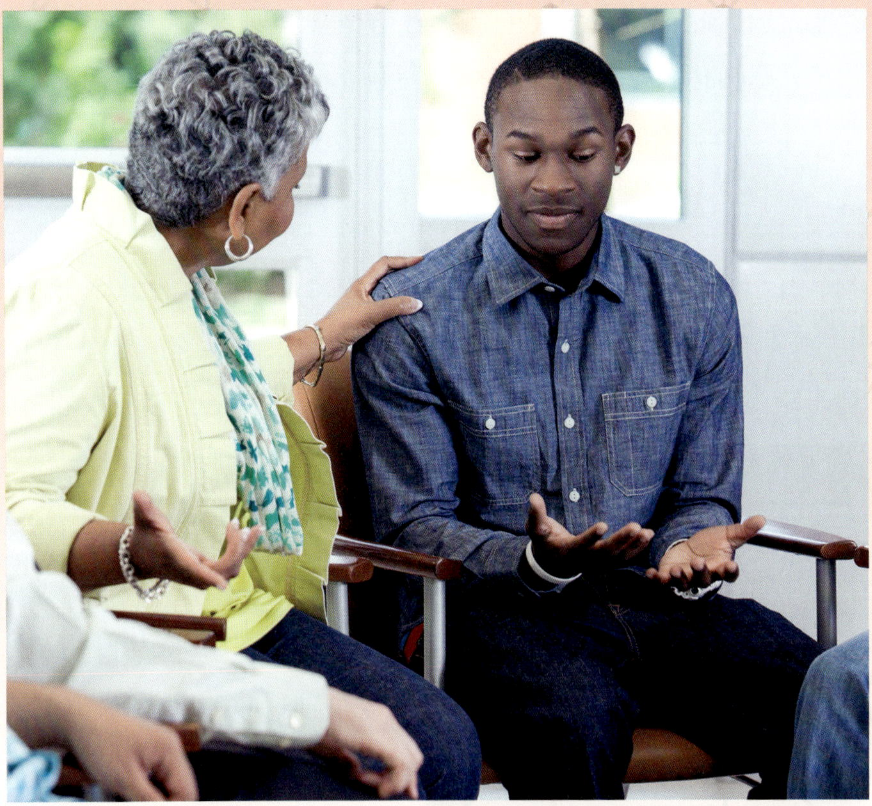

Teens can go to therapy for help managing their depression. Therapists offer ways for patients to alter their moods.

THERAPY FOR DEPRESSION

IPT is a short-term treatment that stems from the idea that depression occurs within one's relationships. Treatment can help teenagers work through the death of a loved one, adapt to changes in relationships, and discuss social isolation. IPT therapists encourage their clients to identify how changes in relationships may alter their mood. A depressed patient in IPT therapy might explore how their family environment and childhood experiences contributed to their depression, and they might learn to acknowledge and move on from traumatic events.

In contrast, cognitive and behavioral therapies focus on how to change harmful thoughts and actions in the present day. Many therapists combine these two approaches and practice cognitive behavioral therapy, or CBT. In CBT, a depressed teen might work with a therapist to recognize overly negative, self-blaming thoughts and replace them with other ways of thinking. The therapist might also give out assignments and homework designed to work at changing behaviors, such as oversleeping or avoiding other people.

Humanistic therapy emphasizes the patient's independence and ability to make decisions. Many therapists practice a blend of approaches, or integrative therapy.

DEPRESSION AND ART

Even during dark, lonely times, depressed people can find comfort and understanding in works of art. For centuries, depressed artists have found ways to channel the pain and numbness of depression into music, literature, and other works of art. The podcast *The Hilarious World of Depression* interviews comedians and other artists who have suffered from depression. In one episode, the podcast's host John Moe asked listeners to share songs that have helped them in hard times. One song came up again and again: "This Year" by the Mountain Goats. The song tells the story of a depressed seventeen-year-old boy, and the refrain repeats, "I'm going to make it through this year if it kills me." John Darnielle, the lead singer and songwriter of the Mountain Goats, was a depressed teen who went through many difficult years. The song was inspired by memories of his seventeen-year-old self.

Some therapists also run group therapy sessions for small groups of patients who struggle with similar symptoms.

Going to therapy can be an intimidating experience. Telling secrets to a stranger is no small task. But therapists will work hard to make patients feel comfortable and address any concerns. As clinical psychologist Loren Soeiro explains, "When you're in therapy, you don't have to talk the whole time. You don't have to talk at all, if you're not up for it. It's your time."[33] Soeiro explains that a good therapist's job is to empathize with clients and help them accept their own feelings. "You should get the sense that he or she can feel what you feel, and understands what it's like to be you," Soeiro told BuzzFeed.[34] Allyson L. shared her experience of therapy with Sarah Schuster on the Mighty. "It can be extremely painful at times and you may feel really bad for a few days reflecting on what was brought to the surface," Allyson wrote, "but then you'll learn how to heal correctly."[35]

> "You should get the sense that your [therapist] can feel what you feel, and understands what it's like to be you."[34]
>
> *—Loren Soeiro, clinical psychologist*

It can be more difficult for teens under eighteen to seek out medical treatment for depression. Teens may worry that their parents will not support them or understand their illness: "It can be hard for teens to access mental health resources because they don't want to tell their parents about their problem,"[36] said Dr. Michele Kerulis, a licensed counselor and professor at the Family Institute at Northwestern. However, it is possible for underage teens to seek out therapy on their own. School counselors can offer sessions and direct students to free or affordable counseling options. Rachel Kazez, a social worker from Chicago, started a company called All Along when she saw a need for accessible information about how to pay for therapy. She helps people navigate therapy offerings in their area and understand how to use insurance to help pay for treatment. In 2017, writer Crissy Milazzo created a free spreadsheet of affordable therapy options across the United States, helping therapy-seekers look for options in their area.

Not all teens benefit from therapy for depression. Some may find they don't respond to therapy at all; others may experience some improvement but still struggle daily with depression symptoms. Experts recommend therapy as a treatment option for mild and moderate depression, but they warn that it may not be enough for teens who are suffering from severe depression.

ANTIDEPRESSANT MEDICATIONS

Antidepressant medications, also known as antidepressants, typically come in pill form and are taken daily. There are several different types of antidepressants. The most popular

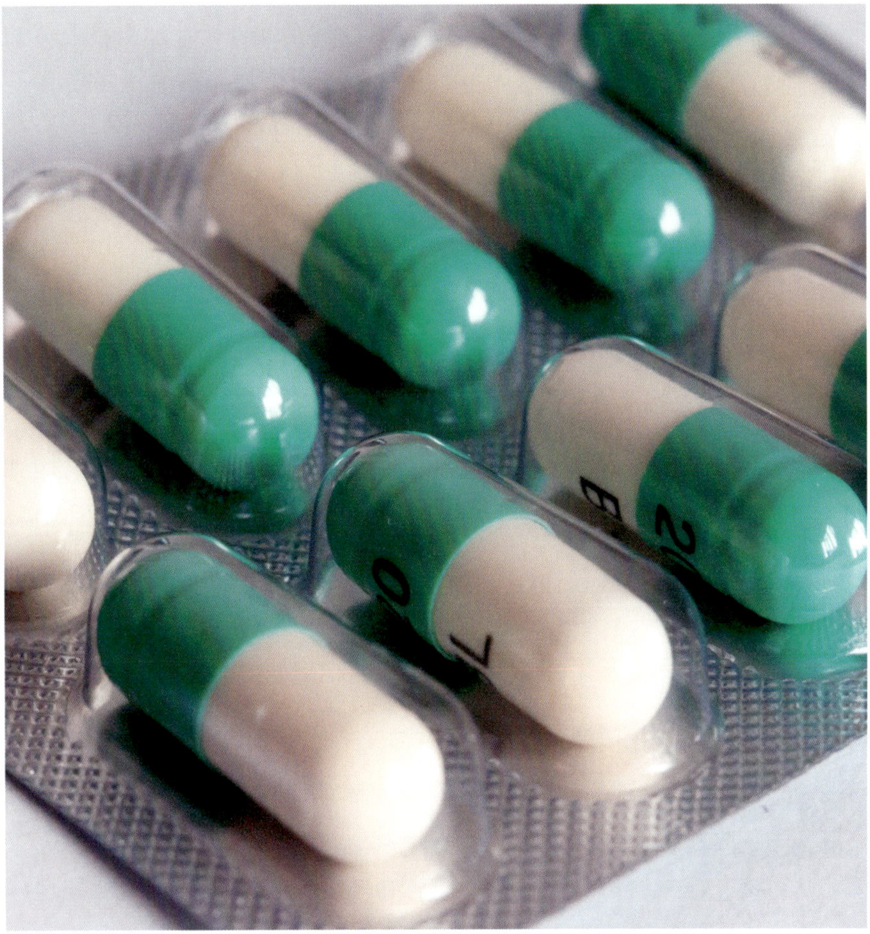

Some people with depression are prescribed antidepressants. Antidepressants do not work for everyone.

antidepressants are called selective serotonin reuptake inhibitors (SSRIs). SSRIs approved by the Food and Drug Administration (FDA) for adolescents are Lexapro, Prozac, and Symbyax. SSRIs work by keeping the brain from reabsorbing a neurotransmitter called serotonin. This action processes more serotonin in the brain, where it's believed to help lift mood and energy. About 60 to 70 percent of depressed patients are helped by antidepressants. But most antidepressants were developed and tested with adult patients in mind, which means they may work differently for teens.

Most antidepressants tend to have relatively mild side effects. Side effects of SSRIs include headache, nausea, diarrhea, and some weight loss or gain. However, there is a risk that taking antidepressants can increase the risk of suicidal ideation. An FDA research review showed that children and teens with mental illness who took antidepressants were more likely to think about suicide than children and teens who did not.

Many depressed teens feel helped by antidepressants, even when they struggle against the stigma of taking a pill for a mental disorder. An anonymous woman who started taking antidepressants at sixteen shared her experiences with *New York* magazine. "There are two big misconceptions about taking antidepressants: that you'll turn into a zombie, and that you're weak for being on them," she wrote. "I'm guilty of still believing that second one, and it's my biggest struggle with antidepressants."[37]

> **"There are two big misconceptions about taking antidepressants: that you'll turn into a zombie, and that you're weak for being on them."[37]**
>
> ***—Anonymous woman***

Since depression can have multiple causes, it makes sense there are many equally valid options for treating the disorder. Depressed teens can

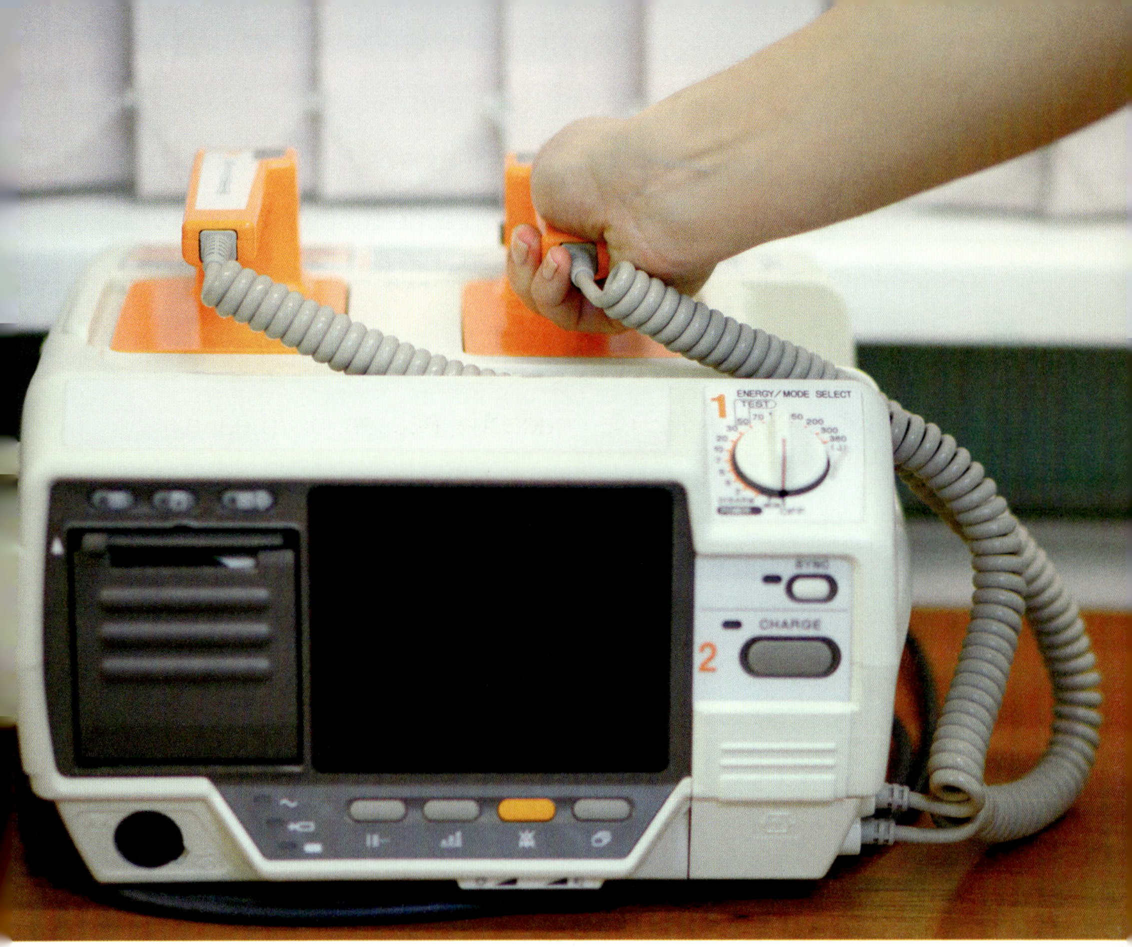

ECT developed from electroshock therapy. It is known to stimulate the brain and help treat depression.

choose to combine therapy and antidepressants or to use both at different times over the course of treatment. Good mental health care professionals work with each patient to find the best treatment plan for each individual. It is important to only take prescribed medication as directed by a mental health care professional.

ECT AND KETAMINE THERAPIES

Two less common depression treatments, electroconvulsive therapy (ECT) and ketamine treatments, may also be effective for depressed teens. ECT, formerly called electroshock therapy, was invented in the late 1930s. In ECT, mental health professionals send electric shocks directly to the brain, intentionally causing a seizure. ECT advocates believe that the seizures help the brain send stronger chemical signals in the nervous system, which corrects damages in the hormone system. While the treatment worked well in some cases, it often had serious side effects, such as short-term memory loss. As time went on, doctors and researchers improved the ECT process to minimize risks. A 2016 study in the *Journal of Child and Adolescent Psychopharmacology* found that more than three-fourths of teen patients who were studied responded well to ECT.

Ketamine is an anesthetic, or pain-numbing drug. It can also make people high and cause hallucinations. Some researchers believe it also has potential as a powerful antidepressant. A 2018 study in the *Journal of Child and Adolescent Psychopharmacology* tested the effects of ketamine on teens with treatment-resistant depression. Treatment-resistant depression is depression that has not improved even after medical treatments. The study found that five of the thirteen participants had a significant positive response, a result the researchers said was promising.

In 2018, researchers at the University of Utah began studying a potential new treatment for depression. The researchers were

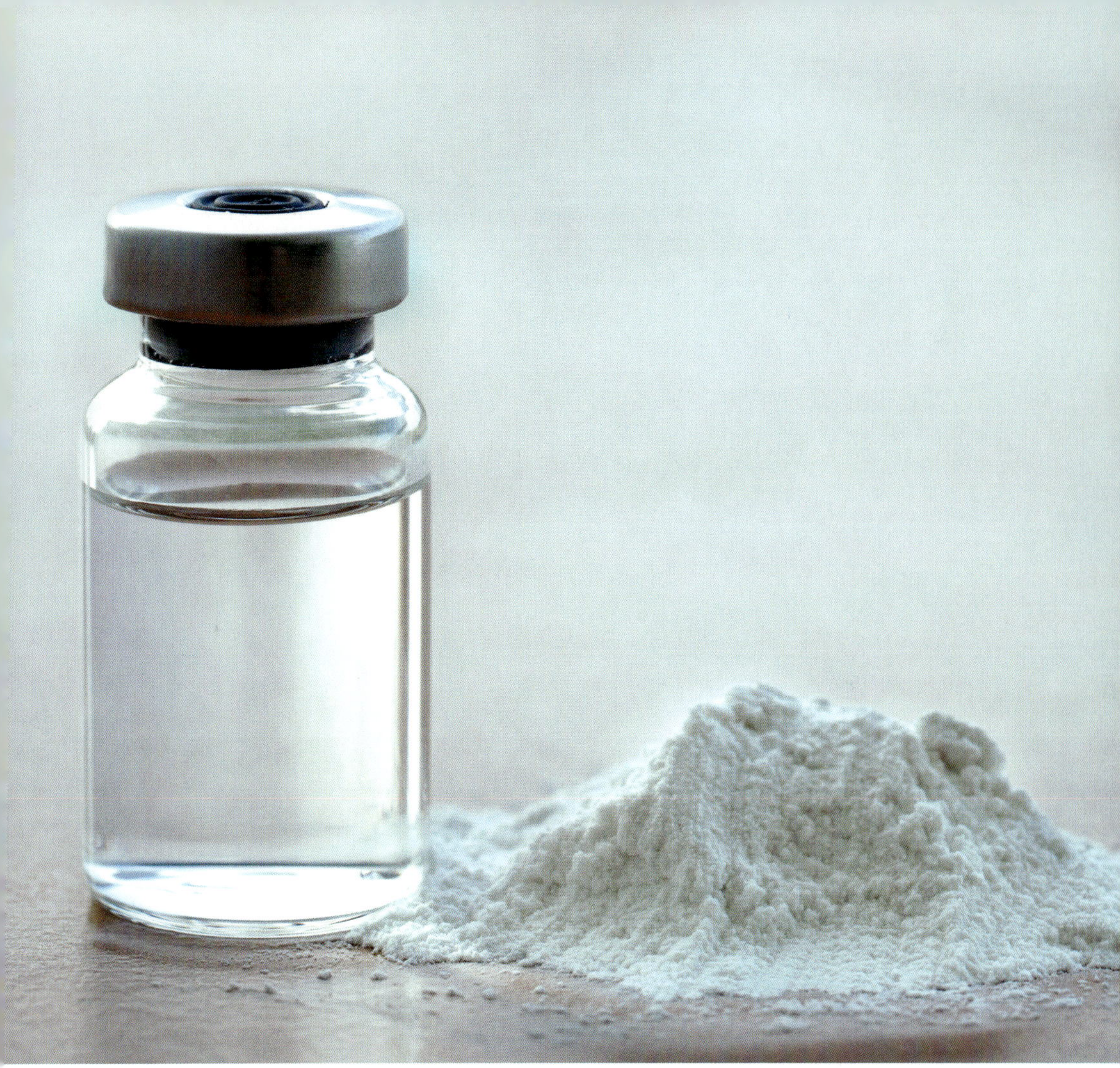

Ketamine is an anesthetic. It is typically used to help chronic pain, but some researchers believe it also helps depression.

curious about the effects of anesthetic drugs, or types of drugs used to dull pain and make people unconscious. They had seen evidence that these drugs could change the way the brain worked, and they wondered if an anesthetic could help treat depression. The researchers found ten volunteers who had depression and had not been successfully treated with antidepressants. The youngest participant was eighteen years

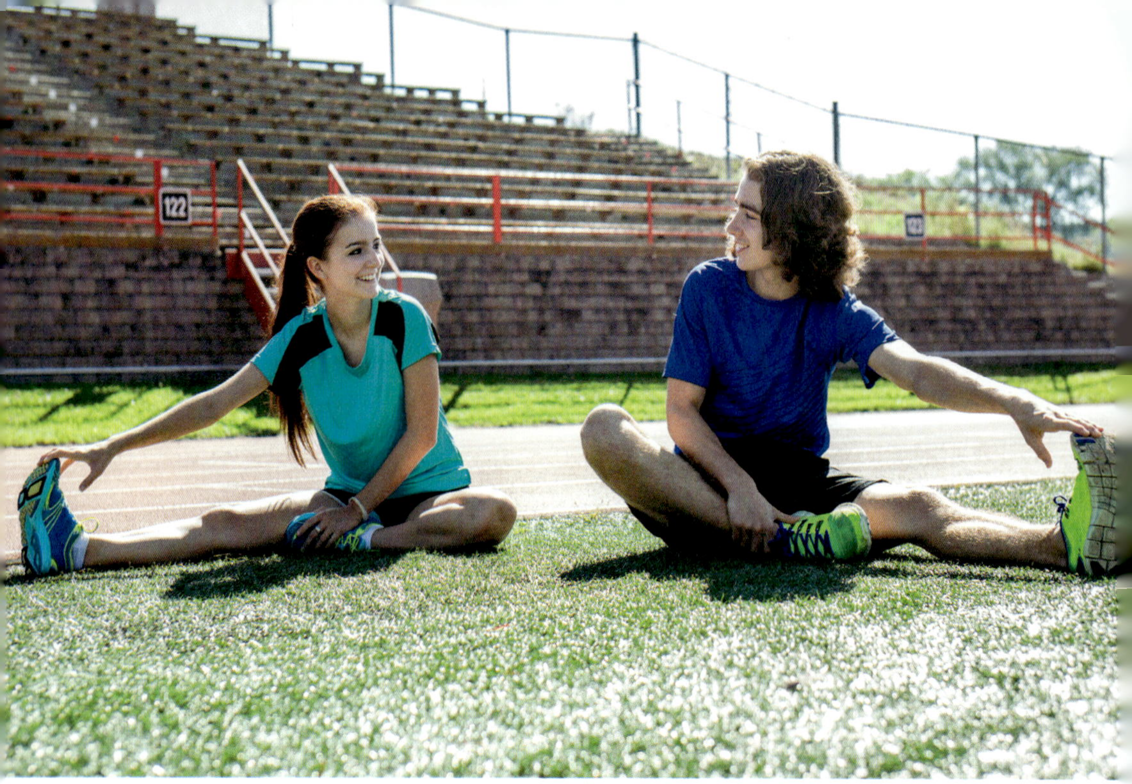

Regular exercise often improves mood. It may give some people more energy and self-confidence.

old. Each participant received a high dose of an anesthetic called propofol. The dose made each participant deeply sedated, with significantly slowed brain activity, for about fifteen minutes. The researchers repeated this practice over several sessions. They found that six of the ten participants saw significant improvement in their depression symptoms. The researchers recommended more research into this potential depression treatment.

EXERCISE AND SELF-CARE

Getting medical treatment for depression is only part of the battle. Teens must also figure out how to manage their symptoms in regular life. Lifestyle adjustments can be difficult to make, but they can also ease the smaller day-to-day battles of living with depression. One common piece of advice for depressed people is to exercise regularly. Exercise might lift someone's mood, energy, and self-esteem. According to a research review by Dr. Nandini Mani, there is some truth to this advice for depressed teens. Mani looked at multiple studies of the effect of exercise on teen depression and concluded that exercise "appears to be a strategy with modest benefits and little downside."[38] In other words, exercise may help with depression, and it probably won't hurt.

Adults who have survived teen depression advocate for self-care, or taking time to treat oneself with kindness and respect for one's needs. Rhea Butcher is a nonbinary comedian who uses the pronouns *they* and *them*. Butcher suffered from anxiety and depression as a teen and young adult. "When I was my most depressed, I would deprive myself from everything," they remember.[39] When asked what they would tell their younger self about dealing with depression, Butcher advises, "Get up and try making your bed . . . and, like, make sure you drink water."[40] These simple acts of caring for the self can help keep low moods from becoming too extreme. Butcher also cares for themself by practicing a self-awareness technique called HALT. When they become

"Get up and try making your bed . . . and, like, make sure you drink water."[40]

—Rhea Butcher, comedian

MENTAL HEALTH FIRST AID

It can be hard to see an acquaintance or stranger go through a mental health crisis and not know whether or how to help. Mental Health First Aid is an organization that teaches people to recognize and help with mental health emergencies. The organization is run by the National Council for Behavioral Health and the Missouri Department of Mental Health. It offers one-day workshops similar to CPR certification courses. Workshops teach participants how to recognize the symptoms of mental health crises. For example, the workshop helps people look for signs that a person they know is at increased risk of suicide or self-harm. That way, participants feel more empowered to make decisions about whether and when to reach out for emergency help. The workshops help people explore their thoughts about mental illness and break down some of the harmful or inaccurate ideas they may have about conditions such as depression. Mental Health First Aid offers workshops specifically for teens.

upset, they ask themself if they are Hungry, Angry, Lonely, or Tired. Then, they try to meet whatever needs they sense.

MENTAL HEALTH RESOURCES AND EDUCATION

There is help available for teens in a mental health crisis. The National Alliance on Mental Illness (NAMI) and the Anxiety and Depression Association of America (AADA) offer information and advocacy for people with mental illnesses like depression. The National Suicide Prevention Lifeline offers help around the clock, as does the Trevor Project (1-866-488-7386), a national suicide hotline for LGBTQ youth. The National Institute of Mental Health (NIMH) is a valuable

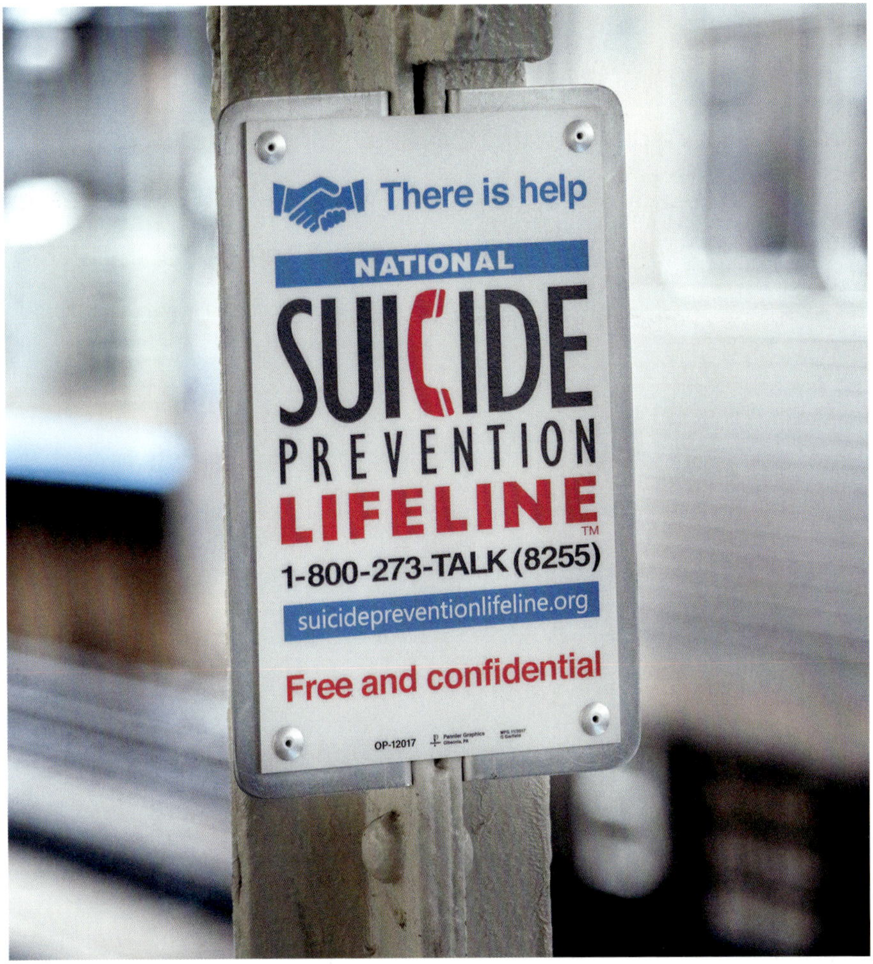
There is help
NATIONAL
SUICIDE
PREVENTION
LIFELINE
1-800-273-TALK (8255)
suicidepreventionlifeline.org
Free and confidential

Depression can cause suicidal thoughts. There are many help centers to call if someone is contemplating suicide.

resource for mental health research, and *Teen Vogue* and BuzzFeed both offer high-quality online journalism on teen mental health issues.

Other organizations are looking for new ways to help teens recognize the symptoms of depression as early as possible. In 2018, the American Academy of Pediatrics (AAP) announced that it had updated its guidelines on identifying and treating teen depression. The AAP stated that it would start educating pediatricians on how to screen patients for depression and come up with a treatment plan. "We would like to see teens fill out a depression screening tool as a routine part of their regular wellness visit," said Dr. Amy Cheung, one of the guidelines' authors.[41]

These resources are also vital for family and friends of depressed teens. Sometimes the loved ones of depressed people feel like they should be doing more to help. But just as someone wouldn't try to perform surgery on a friend with a broken bone, it's not any friend's job to try to treat another person's depression. People with depression benefit greatly from having friends and allies who can give them love and support. Mental health treatment is a job for mental health professionals.

Johns Hopkins University's Adolescent Depression Awareness Program (ADAP) is looking to expand mental health education in US schools. The program is a three-hour set of lessons designed for teaching in schools. The developers of ADAP hope to improve teenagers' ability to recognize and talk about depression. ADAP also offers guides for teachers and parents on the signs of teen depression. The University of Illinois is developing a phone app, BiAffect, to use data and fitness trackers to guess if users are depressed. One of the

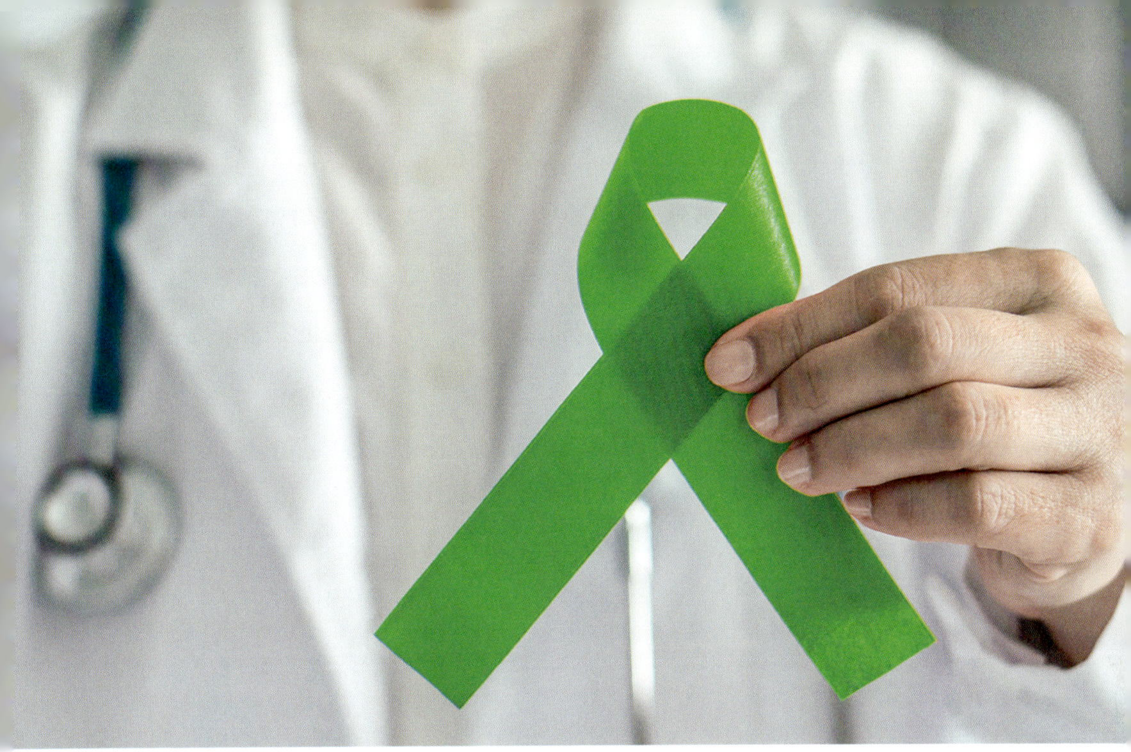

Green ribbons symbolize mental health awareness. World Mental Health Day is observed on October 10 every year.

developers, Dr. Alex Loew, said, "The goal of our work aims to turn smartphones into 'fitness trackers' for the human brain."[42]

October 10 is World Mental Health Day. It's an opportunity for people around the world to share their stories of mental illness and recovery, to support others undergoing health crises, and to chip away at the stigma that still surrounds mental illness and treatment. On World Mental Health Day 2019, people from around the world shared their stories online and used the hashtag #WorldMentalHealthDay. Their combined voices reminded everyone who struggles with depression that there is hope and that they are not alone.

SOURCE NOTES

INTRODUCTION: THE NAMELESS PROBLEM

1. Naomi Ekperigin and John Moe, "Naomi Ekperigin Brings in Her Baggage, Unpacks It," *Hilarious World of Depression*, December 9, 2018. www.hilariousworld.org.

2. Ekperigin and Moe, "Naomi Ekperigin Brings in Her Baggage, Unpacks It."

3. Ekperigin and Moe, "Naomi Ekperigin Brings in Her Baggage, Unpacks It."

4. Ekperigin and Moe, "Naomi Ekperigin Brings in Her Baggage, Unpacks It."

5. Ekperigin and Moe, "Naomi Ekperigin Brings in Her Baggage, Unpacks It."

6. Ekperigin and Moe, "Naomi Ekperigin Brings in Her Baggage, Unpacks It."

CHAPTER 1: WHAT IS TEEN DEPRESSION?

7. Elise Jamison, "This Is What Depression Really Feels Like," *HuffPost*, March 2, 2014. www.huffpost.com.

8. Francis M. Mondimore and Patrick Kelly, *Adolescent Depression: A Guide for Parents*. Baltimore: Johns Hopkins University Press, 2015, p. 23.

9. *Diagnostic and Statistical Manual of Mental Disorders (DSM-5).* Washington, DC: American Psychiatric Association Publishing, 2013, p. 169.

10. "What Causes Depression?" *Harvard Health Publishing*, June 24, 2019. www.health.harvard.edu.

11. Kurt Kroenke, "PHQ-9 (Patient Health Questionnaire-9)," *MDCalc*, n.d. www.mdcalc.com.

12. Maria Shadrina et al., "Genetics Factors in Major Depression Disease," *Front Psychiatry*, July 23, 2018. www.ncbi.nlm.nih.gov.

13. Quoted in Michael Baggs and Christian Hewgill, "LGBT Mental Health: 'Being the Butt of Gay Jokes Made Me Ill,'" *BBC News*, November 8, 2018. www.bbc.com.

14. Quoted in Susanna Schrobsdorff, "Teen Depression and Anxiety: Why the Kids Are Not Alright," *Time*, October 27, 2016. www.time.com.

CHAPTER 2: HOW DOES DEPRESSION AFFECT TEENS?

15. Morgan Parker, *Who Put This Song On?* New York: Delacorte Press, 2019.

16. Brynn, "Overcoming Teen Depression and Anxiety: Brynn's Story," *Your Teen*, n.d. yourteenmag.com.

17. Quoted in Patti Harrison and John Moe, "Patti Harrison Figures Out Who She Is and She's a Woman Who Likes Gross Jokes," *Hilarious World of Depression*, November 6, 2017. www.hilariousworld.org.

18. Quoted in Andrea Park, "Cara Delevingne Opens Up About Battling Depression and Suicidal Thoughts as a Teenager," *W*, September 29, 2017. www.wmagazine.com.

19. Erika Wenzel, "When Teenage Heartbreak Turns Into Depression," *The Mighty*, July 9, 2015. www.themighty.com.

20. Quoted in Dan Vergano, "Was It a Drug Overdose, or a Suicide?" *BuzzFeed*, July 18, 2018. www.buzzfeednews.com.

21. Quoted in Melissa Healy, "Suicide Rates for U.S. Teens and Young Adults Are the Highest on Record," *Los Angeles Times*, June 18, 2019. www.latimes.com.

22. Harrison and Moe, "Patti Harrison Figures Out Who She Is and She's a Woman Who Likes Gross Jokes."

CHAPTER 3: HOW DOES TEEN DEPRESSION AFFECT SOCIETY?

23. "A Letter to . . . My Sister, Who Has Conquered Her Depression," *The Guardian*, December 23, 2017. www.theguardian.com.

SOURCE NOTES CONTINUED

24. Nicola Morgan, "How Can Teenagers Help a Friend with Mental Illness?" *Nicola Morgan*, July 12, 2016. www.nicolamorgan.com.

25. Quoted in Brett Sholtis, "'There Are No Answers': One Family Pushes Forward after Losing Teenager to Suicide," *PA Post*, January 3, 2012. www.papost.org.

26. Carl, "Anxiety and Depression Took Over My Life," *Time to Change*, July 1, 2017. www.time-to-change.org.uk.

27. Quoted in John Otis "She Lost Years to Addiction and Depression. Now 54, She Has Work to Do," *New York Times*, December 28, 2016. www.nytimes.com.

28. Quoted in Linda Carroll, "Teen's Story of Depression Goes Viral," *Today*, October 8, 2013. www.today.com.

29. Quoted in Allison Abrams, "Why We Need to Stop Demonizing Antidepressants," *Psychology Today*. June 8, 2018. www.psychologytoday.com.

30. Prachi Gupta, "Stories About My Brother," *Jezebel*, September 26, 2019. www.jezebel.com.

31. Gupta, "Stories About My Brother."

32. Quoted in Gupta, "Stories About My Brother."

CHAPTER 4: HOW CAN WE TREAT AND PREVENT TEEN DEPRESSION?

33. Quoted in Sally Tamarkin, "3 Therapists Describe WTF Therapy Is Actually Like," *BuzzFeed*, October 3, 2017. www.buzzfeed.com.

34. Quoted in Tamarkin, "3 Therapists Describe WTF Therapy Is Actually Like."

35. Quoted in Sarah Schuster, "The Advice No One Tells You About Going to Therapy," *The Mighty*, February 16, 2017. www.themighty.com.

36. Quoted in Helaina Hovitz, "Mental Health Resources to Know if You Identify as LGBTQ," *Teen Vogue*, June 1, 2017. www.teenvogue.com.

37. Quoted in Tessa Miller, "9 Women on Their Experiences with Antidepressants," *The Cut*, January 9, 2018. www.thecut.com.

38. Nandini Mani, "Can Exercise Help Relieve Teen Depression?" *Harvard Health Publishing*, August 10, 2016. www.health.harvard.edu.

39. Rhea Butcher, Dave Ross, and Hampton Yount, "Interview with Rhea Butcher," *Suicide Buddies*, September 26, 2019. https://starburns.audio.

40. Butcher, Ross, and Yount, "Interview with Rhea Butcher."

41. Quoted in "American Academy of Pediatrics Publishes Teen Depression Guidelines that Equip Physicians to Tackle Mental Health Issues," *American Academy of Pediatrics*, February 26, 2018. www.aap.org.

42. Quoted in Lilly Dancyger, "Could Smartphone Apps Help Curb Teen Depression?" *Rolling Stone*, January 8, 2019. www.rollingstone.com.

FOR FURTHER RESEARCH

BOOKS

Andrea Balinson, *Depression, Anxiety, and Bipolar Disorders*. Broomall, PA: Mason Crest, 2018.

Megan A. Moreno and Ana Radovic, eds., *Technology and Adolescent Mental Health*. New York: Springer Science+Business Media, 2018.

Don Nardo, *Teen Guide to Mental Health*. San Diego, CA: ReferencePoint Press, 2020.

Peggy J. Parks, *Kids and Mental Illness*. San Diego, CA: ReferencePoint Press, 2019.

Jan Scott and Mary J. Tacchi, *Depression: A Very Short Introduction*. Oxford, UK: Oxford University Press, 2017.

INTERNET SOURCES

Adryan Corcione, "How to Find a Therapist When Your Parents Won't Help," *Teen Vogue*, August 29, 2017. www.teenvogue.com.

"Screening for Depression," *Anxiety and Depression Association of America*, n.d. www.adaa.org.

Melinda Smith et al., "Helping Someone with Depression," *HelpGuide*, October 2019. www.helpguide.org.

WEBSITES

National Alliance on Mental Illness
www.nami.org/find-support/teens-and-young-adults

The National Alliance on Mental Illness offers support and resources for teens who are looking to help themselves, a friend, or a loved one with depression.

National Institute of Mental Health
www.nimh.nih.gov/health/publications/teen-depression/index.shtml

The National Institute of Mental Health offers a guide for teens on recognizing, understanding, and dealing with depression.

National Suicide Prevention Lifeline
https://suicidepreventionlifeline.org

The National Suicide Prevention Lifeline is available around the clock for anyone who is struggling with suicidal thoughts or needs someone to talk to in a difficult time.

INDEX

INDEX CONTINUED

IMAGE CREDITS

Cover: © Krakenimages.com/Shutterstock Images
5: © mimagephotography/Shutterstock Images
9: © February_Love/Shutterstock Images
13: © Voyagerix/Shutterstock Images
15: © Everett Historical/Shutterstock Images
16: © Kzenon/Shutterstock Images
19: © SDI Productions/iStockphoto
20: © Motortion Films/Shutterstock Images
27: © Estrada Anton/Shutterstock Images
31: © Kzenon/Shutterstock Images
33: © Twocoms/Shutterstock Images
34: © LightField Studios/Shutterstock Images
39: © Sami Sert/iStockphoto
40: © Wollertz/Shutterstock Images
43: © Antonio Guillem/Shutterstock Images
46: © alejandrophotography/iStockphoto
48: © smolaw/Shutterstock Images
51: © SpeedKingz/Shutterstock Images
55: © SDI Productions/iStockphoto
59: © callumrc/Shutterstock Images
61: © Pavel L Photo and Video/Shutterstock Images
63: © Pcess609/Shutterstock Images
64: © Lopolo/Shutterstock Images
67: © ventdusud/iStockphoto
69: © Chinnapong/Shutterstock Images

ABOUT THE AUTHOR

A.W. Buckey is a writer and pet-sitter living in Brooklyn, New York.